TALK TO ME

Sharing the extraordinary stories of ten everyday people engaging in psychotherapy, this book takes the reader into the room, showing the realities of being in therapy and providing insight into the perspectives of both the patient and the clinician.

Through these cases from her own practice, author and psychotherapist Bianca Denny dissects, unravels and reconstructs experiences of grief, denial, jealousy, shame, desire, and letting go. A terminally ill woman desperate to reconcile with her estranged family. A new mother on the precipice of admission to a psychiatric unit. A delusional man, intent on harming his wife. A bachelor who self-sabotages his last chance of happiness. An adult daughter struggling to understand the relationship with her mother, in the wake of her parents' divorce. A person for whom a diagnosis of ADHD raises more questions than it answers. Denny shares her personal and professional insight through reactions of vulnerability, sadness, compassion and frustration. Readers are invited into the minds of patients as well as the internal workings of a therapist's mind.

Exploring the complexity of the patient and therapist relationship, and what actually happens in therapy, this book is essential reading for qualifying and early career therapists.

Bianca Denny is a clinical psychologist, working in private practice in Melbourne, Australia. She is an accredited supervisor of trainee (provisional) psychologists and those seeking clinical endorsement. Bianca also contributes to the media, writing on mental health and psychology topics.

TALK TO ME

Lessons from Patients and Their Therapist

BIANCA DENNY

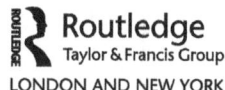

Routledge
Taylor & Francis Group

LONDON AND NEW YORK

Designed cover image: Getty Images

First published 2026
by Routledge
4 Park Square, Milton Park, Abingdon, Oxon OX14 4RN

and by Routledge
605 Third Avenue, New York, NY 10158

Routledge is an imprint of the Taylor & Francis Group, an informa business

British Library Cataloguing-in-Publication Data
A catalogue record for this book is available from the British Library

ISBN: 978-1-041-02966-3 (hbk)
ISBN: 978-1-041-02965-6 (pbk)
ISBN: 978-1-003-62164-5 (ebk)

DOI: 10.4324/9781003621645

Typeset in Dante and Avenir
by Apex CoVantage, LLC

For Emma and James

CONTENTS

Acknowledgements   ix

   Introduction   1

1 Synchronicity   7

2 Wash, rinse, repeat   19

3 Peter Perfect   31

4 Is my therapist annoyed at me?   39

5 Death becomes her   49

6 The human condition   59

7 Similarity   65

8 The unsent letter   73

9 All work and no play   83

10 Jealousy is a curse   93

Index   103

ACKNOWLEDGEMENTS

Nothing can be achieved without the help of others. Throughout my studies and work I have benefited greatly from professional and personal mentoring and support.

Graeme Gibbons, for constructive feedback on this manuscript, but moreover for teaching me the value of relational therapy and the restorative power of care. The question of 'where are you in this?' transformed my writing and work as a therapist.
Laura Baldwin and Elena Bhattacharya, for reminding me that I can do difficult things.
Catherine Deveny and the Gunnas community, for your kindness, perpetual enthusiasm, and unwavering encouragement. Special thanks to Carol Sandiford.
Brett Faubert and Cassandra Rutherford, for listening.
Susana Gavidia-Payne, for comments and guidance on the introductory chapter.
Richard Inglis, for feedback on several chapters, and our discussions around the concept of this book.

My children, Emma and James.

Last, my patients – past, present, and future. Thank you for entrusting me with your stories, and for allowing me to share in your lives, through good times and bad.

Thanks also to Dr Alisoun Gardner-Medwin, daughter of Helena Shire, for permission to reproduce 'I was the wrong music' by Olive Fraser, from *The Wrong Music: The Poems of Olive Fraser; 1909–1977*, edited by Helena Mennie Shire (Canongate, 1989).

INTRODUCTION

"Whatever happens," a therapist once said to me at a time when my life was very much at sea, "I'll be here for you." And they were.

As a therapy patient, the most valuable offerings have not been a label or name for my experiences, nor the use of jargon or terminology to explain that which ails me. At times when my world has seemed a dark and conniving place, therapy has offered respite, sanctuary, safety, and security.

As a therapist, I most often sit on the other side of the couch. I have the privilege of listening to people tell their stories, exploring with them the twists and turns of their lives, aiding in organising and understanding the culmination of their experiences.

Every individual has a story, and every story is unique. But while patients differ in the details of their lives, the human experience shows us to be more similar than different. Several core attributes typify this, including: the search for meaning and purpose, the importance of attachment to caregivers and loved ones, the compulsion for connection with others, the pain and grief of loss, the inevitability of death, the quest for forgiveness and healing, and a broad spectrum of feelings ranging from melancholia to euphoria. Mostly, we want to understand and be understood.

But in today's culture, listening and understanding seem to have given way to a desire for quick-fixes of all things that worry us. Diagnosis and medication are increasingly emphasised as a panacea for life's woes. We look to TikTok 'experts' for 30-second answers to fundamental questions and existential queries. Motivational quotes are liked and loved and shared with wild abandon. Ex-partners are readily labelled narcissistic or socio-pathic. A well-organised pantry is extrapolated to a diagnosis of obsessive-compulsive disorder. Distraction and inattention are deemed to be ADHD and medicated accordingly.

With better advocacy and public awareness around psychological wellbeing, patients are increasingly presenting not with curiosity about symptoms and experiences, but instead more commonly seeking absolute answers and, for some, confirmation of self-diagnosis. Armchair experts on social media seem to fuel the collective appetite for the explanation and categorisation of every quirk and characteristic, whether innocuous or pathological. Algorithms have become the modern version of a self-fulfilling prophecy: scroll and you

DOI: 10.4324/9781003621645-1

shall find. But the medicalisation of human experiences provides scant opportunity to sit with distress, to grow through it, or to grow with it. Rather, there is a rush to explain, to label, to treat. We are quick to diagnose and fast to medicate. But preoccupation with diagnosis can distract from core aspects of the human experience, guarding against being fully present with a person and their experience. Most often, a diagnosis is the least interesting thing about a person.

I trained as a clinical psychologist. Diagnosis of mental disorders was the primary focus of years of study. My crumpled, dog-eared copy of the *Diagnostic and Statistical Manual (DSM)* bears witness to this. But as I moved away from assessment and further into work as a therapist, I began to hear more stories from people whose experiences failed to fit neatly into a diagnostic category, or whose trajectory or outcomes in life could not be easily explained by a bunch of criteria and diagnostic specifiers. Diagnosis and diagnostic language do, of course, remain useful. It provides a communication tool between professionals, and assists many people in understanding their experiences. But the notion of 'concept creep' and the increasing application of labels and terms to normal human experiences pathologises rather than acknowledges the breadth of human experiences and behaviours.

Therapy provides an antidote to this need to explain away individuals' quirks and characteristics. A place in which the many and varied experiences of the human condition can be expressed and explored. An opportunity to slow down, to unfurl, to sit with and tolerate the trials and tribulations inherent to life.

For many, therapy remains a curious concept. How exactly does talking therapy work? How does it differ from a chat with a friend? People who may benefit from therapy are sometimes reluctant to participate, perhaps trepidatious about what to expect, and understandably nervous about introspection and what it may bring. I hope this book will give some clarity around this, encouraging a broader idea about what the process may look like and what value can be derived from it.

Historically, mental illness has been poorly understood. Treatment ranged from well-intentioned, dangerous, to outright cruel. Public perception was shaped by cultural touchstones such as Freud's ubiquitous couch and Nurse Ratched doling out medication in *One Flew Over the Cuckoo's Nest*. Mental health treatment was once reserved for people at opposite ends of the psychological spectrum: at one end, the wealthy, privileged (and arguably neurotic) subset of the population who had the time and money to engage in treatment; at the other, severely unwell patients with unremitting symptoms, perhaps housed in an asylum or institution.

Coming to the present time, improved understanding of the biological and environmental (nature and nurture, respectively) precipitants to mental illness has led to a marked change in societal perception of mental health and mental illness.[1] Now, most people experiencing mental illness live in the community, accessing care through private providers or outpatient services. Recovery is not only possible, but endorsed and supported in both professional and social contexts. Advocacy and understanding around mental health have led to reduced stigma around help-seeking, hence informing a surge in the popularity of therapy.

Therapy represents advocacy for a focus on the self and the factors and experiences that have brought an individual to the current juncture of their life. Within this milieu is the opportunity to gain insight, and, if desired, instigate change. The true value of therapy comes not from dispensing advice or labels; effective therapy prompts curiosity and reflection rather than a focus on basic end goals. Care is always the cure.

Therapists encourage patients to ask questions of themselves, and seek to support an exploration of patients' understanding of their world:

Where am I in this?

How did I find myself mixed up in this situation?

What attracted me to this person, who has now caused me such harm?

Which parts of my self and my history may have predisposed me to being in this relationship or finding myself in this difficult situation?

Have I experienced this pattern before? Perhaps with other people, in previous relationships, at other workplaces, or in other social settings?

Here, we resist the temptation to wholly externalise or blame others for our problems. We turn away from focusing on others' behaviour, being mindful to not engage in speculative activity of trying to 'figure someone out'. Seeking to understand the impetus for another's actions often leads to inferred conclusions or blanket statements drawn without evidence; for example, my ex-partner's behaviour is unacceptable to me, no one in their right mind could treat another person like that, only a narcissist could act in that way, they *must* have narcissistic personality disorder. Engaging in this style of derivative thinking and focusing on others' behaviour can satisfy curiosity and bolster our own ego, but presents little scope for meaningful action. Seeking to modify another person's behaviour – with or without their knowledge – invariably leads to frustration for both parties.

PSYCHOTHERAPY ENCOUNTERS

A range of human experiences and psychological phenomena are elucidated in this book. It adopts a humanistic perspective, in which relationships, connection, and positive regard are emphasised.

Each of the ten chapters tells the tale of a psychotherapy encounter between myself and a patient. Specific psychological concepts are illustrated through each encounter. The chapters may be read sequentially, though each chapter stands on its own.

A story is not simply told, it is also heard. There are (at least) two people in a therapy room: the patient and the therapist, the orator and the listener. The essential interaction in this relationship – conversations between my patients and me – is explored through ten psychotherapy encounters. Together, patients and I dissect, unravel, and reconstruct experiences of grief, denial, jealousy, shame, desire, and letting go. These stories epitomise the human condition. This is the essence of human life, the stuff that makes us tick, the mess that drives us mad.

- John, whose childhood experiences of deprivation and loss are compounded by more recent experiences of grief.
- Luke, whose tendency towards repetition compulsion and self-sabotage make for a complex therapeutic relationship.
- Hannah, whose denial about the state of her relationship illustrates both the adaptive and maladaptive aspects of defence mechanisms.
- Isabelle, pregnant with her first child and on the precipice of an admission to a psychiatric hospital, vexes me with her adoration of her psychiatrist, bringing issues of countertransference to the fore.
- Lee, a terminally ill patient whose existential dread uncovers dark family secrets.
- Chris, whose recent ADHD diagnosis is not the panacea they were expecting.
- Maya, who is more similar to her mother than she may care to admit.
- Jo, whose expressions of distress about her family's dysfunction seem to fall on deaf ears.
- Iliana, whose struggle to find a work-life balance indicates something deeper about her need to belong.
- Finally, the tales of two pathologically jealous men, Nicholas and Brian, shine light on the experiences of both perpetrators and survivors of family violence.

Simultaneously, I learn first-hand that no one is immune to the vicissitudes and challenges of life, not least therapists. Through my own turmoil I come to appreciate the importance of sitting with and exploring my own difficult feelings. I become mindful of my reactions and responses to patients, and realise the impact of my personal experiences on my work as a therapist and the way in which I work with and relate to patients.

Often, we are implored to 'listen hard' or 'listen up' as a way to show attention and gather information. Rather, I hope this book encourages therapists and their patients to speak and listen in a softer way. To sit quietly and move slowly, and in doing so adopt a more open stance that allows us to listen, hear, and, ultimately, understand. Through this, meaningful connection can be established and maintained.

Readers might see aspects of themselves or someone they know within these pages. The clinical vignettes are an amalgamation and extension of true psychotherapy encounters, but have been anonymised and de-identified. No one patient is recognisable in any way.

NOTE

1 The terms *mental health* and *mental illness* are often used interchangeably; in this context *mental health* generally refers to being psychologically well, while *mental illness* refers to the experience of psychological distress or psychiatric illness that impacts a person's capacity to function in areas such as education, employment, social life, and relationships.

FURTHER READING

Bloch, S., & Haslam, N. (2023). *Troubled minds: Understanding and treating mental illness* (rev./updated ed.). Scribe Publications.

Denny, B. (2023, 9 November). Self-diagnosis is on the rise, but is TikTok really to blame? *The Age.*

Diagnostic and statistical manual of mental disorders: DSM-5 (5th ed. Special ed.). (2017). CBS Publishers & Distributors, Pvt. Ltd.

Grosz, S. (2013). *The examined life: How we lose and find ourselves.* Chatto & Windus.

Haslam, N. (2016). Concept creep: Psychology's expanding concepts of harm and pathology. *Psychological Inquiry, 27*(1), 1–17. https://doi.org/10.1080/1047840X.2016.1082418

McWilliams, N. (2011). *Psychoanalytic diagnosis.* Guilford Press.

Rogers, C. R. (2004). *On becoming a person: A therapist's view of psychotherapy.* Constable.

Sperry, L. (2016). *Handbook of diagnosis and treatment of DSM-5 personality disorders: Assessment, case conceptualization, and treatment* (3rd ed.). Routledge.

Surís, A., Holliday, R., & North, C. (2016). The evolution of the classification of psychiatric disorders. *Behavioral Sciences, 6*(1), 5. https://doi.org/10.3390/bs6010005

1

SYNCHRONICITY

Synchronicity is an ever present reality for those have eyes to see it.

Carl Jung

Sometimes reality truly is stranger than fiction. Therapy with John, a man aged in his sixties, was one such instance.

John was an anomaly. Shaggy grey hair, a face creased with layers of deep wrinkles. Perpetually dressed in a uniform of dirty jeans and fleece hooded jumper, whatever the weather. Steel-capped boots, made even more bulky with thick socks.

John would arrive at our sessions in a shiny late-model sports car, providing a stark contrast to his rough appearance. My motor-enthusiast colleague practically salivated at the sound of the car tyres on the gravel; my own jaw dropped upon hearing the starting price of that model of car. John always arrived on the dot of our session time. Never a minute late, never a minute early. He walked at pace across the car park, eyes down, reminiscent of the way one moves when attempting to leave a theatre outside of intermission time.

John settled onto the couch, his bulky frame sinking into the cushions. Distress was etched in his face. Tears hovered on the lower lids of his large blue eyes, soon spilling over onto his cheeks.

His life, he told me, was a mess. The recent dissolution of his marriage – his third and her second – had shattered his world as he knew it. John's adult daughter had urged him to seek help. He openly wondered the purpose of this "talking stuff." Regardless, he needed no convincing or coaxing to speak. John was ready to talk.

John felt betrayed and blindsided by the end of the marriage, which had irrevocably broken down not long after the couple returned from an extensive (and expensive) overseas holiday. John chastised himself for his generosity with finances throughout their relationship. He couldn't help but ponder the coincidence of her departure and the experience of financial problems within his business. His estranged wife refused any contact, with communication now solely through lawyers.

The death of his brother soon after solidified the year as the worst of his life. John recalled the harrowing moment of informing his elderly mother, noting he believed neither he nor his mother would likely recover from his brother's death.

DOI: 10.4324/9781003621645-2

John commented that bad things happen in threes. First, the divorce. Second, business problems. Third, his brother's death. Not in that order, he hastily added, seemingly mindful of how I may perceive his ranking of these adverse life events.

"One, two, three," he stated, counting the numbers on his fingers as if to emphasise his point. A shake of the head signalled disbelief at this terrible string of events.

"Any of those singular events alone would be devastating, but there seems a special cruelty in the compounded impact of the three. It's understandable that you are at such a low ebb, trying to navigate these monumental life events." His response of slowly nodding his head and blinking back tears seemed to confirm his experience of my empathy.

I asked John to share more about his brother. The siblings – four boys in total – were predominantly raised by their mother, with their father leaving the family well before John reached his teen years. John recalled the shock at his father's departure from the family home. There one day, gone the next. No warning, no indication. A vague memory of his father walking out the front door, carrying a suitcase. Their father did not look back at the four wide-eyed boys peering out the front window of the modest council flat. John recalled cajoling his younger brothers away from the window. He closed the door on his mother's bedroom to shield them from the view of her sobbing on the bed. He led the boys to the kitchen and set about preparing a meal.

I reflected to John that this sounded reminiscent of his recent experience with the breakdown of his marriage, with neither his father nor estranged wife looking back as they left. John again nodded, seemingly surprised at the similarities across these events, a realisation of this being more than mere coincidence.

"I still remember, it was tinned beans on toast. We didn't have any butter. The boys wanted butter on their toast, but I couldn't give it to them."

John as a young boy, having just witnessed his father leaving the house, putting aside his own distress to pull together a meal. I silently hypothesised that this task served as a much-needed distraction for John. Unable to save himself and his siblings from the terror of their father leaving the family, he set about accomplishing the task of meeting a more basic need – that of food. John decided in that moment to do all he could to protect his mother and brothers. They had very little, but had each other.

"Always keep a tin of beans in the cupboard, Bianca. You'll never know when you might need them."

I nodded in agreement at his sage advice. "It seems that was a seminal moment in your life. You felt you had to step up. And step up you did."

After our session, I reflected upon John's comments about tinned beans. A scrappy meal, a quick and easy dinner when the cupboards are bare and morale is low. It seemed to be his way of saying, *be prepared – bad things happen, and you need to be ready for them.* I thought of the post-war generation – my grandparents' era – who were notorious for austere financial habits and stockpiling long-life food. This paucity mindset, also known as scarcity mindset, is often associated with individuals being hypervigilant to the prospect of loss and poverty, even in the face of evidence of prosperity or security.

My own grandparents' pantries were full of tinned vegetables and home-made preserves. Not a thing was wasted; lard saved for cooking and baking, seeds dried and planted in the vegetable patch, leftovers served under the auspicious title of 'bubble and squeak'. What we now call organic and environmentally friendly was once the only lifestyle option.

John knew poverty. He knew the value of tinned food, the relative luxury of butter. But most prescient was his memory of the disappointment and despair of not being able to meet his brothers' seemingly simple request for butter. From this, John learned to be prepared. People who have experienced scarcity of resources in their lives (especially around basic needs such as food) often demonstrate a subconscious hypervigilance to protecting against future experiences of paucity. Hence, tinned goods, aversion to waste, a mindset of holding onto things 'just in case'. His precise punctuality and time-keeping in sessions seemed to also be a reflection of this; no time was wasted and he was sure to extract value from sessions.

Moreover, I reflected upon John's reason for telling *me* to keep tinned beans in the cupboard. I wondered if he was looking out for me, caring for me like he cared for his brothers and mother. He had adopted the role of protector from an early age. Was this also playing out in our therapeutic relationship? Did he feel the need to also protect me?

"He completely abandoned us," John continued, detailing that he was left with his mother and siblings in council housing, while John's father and his 'second family' enjoyed wealth and prosperity. John and his family had done what they needed to survive, he stated, with the siblings' petty theft and truancy in adolescence giving way to more serious crime in adulthood. His three siblings spent time in jail for various offences.

I sensed John was downplaying the role of crime in his own life; I imagined there was likely more to his business dealings and bankruptcy than he was sharing. I wondered but did not ask if he had also been imprisoned. As I always tell patients (within the bounds of informed consent and withstanding that no harm against another person is being perpetrated), I am not the police. We are not in an interview room, and therapy is not an interrogation.

My reluctance to probe further on this aspect of John's history may have come from hesitation about rupturing our therapeutic relationship. A rupture represents some kind of fracture or difficulty in the therapeutic relationship. The repair of a therapeutic rupture can be an integral process in therapy, but is typically harder to resolve when occurring very early in treatment, as there has not yet been a chance to establish a strong therapeutic rapport that is integral to repair and resolution of ruptures. During the initial sessions with John I was especially mindful of avoiding rupture, perhaps due to his history of abandonment potentially predisposing him to leaving treatment at the first sign of difficulty in the relationship between us.

The role of money in John's life was a slippery topic. Similar to my queries regarding criminal behaviour, I was concerned that raising it might rupture our therapeutic relationship. Questioning his honesty around money may cause him to shut down sharing other aspects of his life. An expensive car, international travel – this was at odds with his stated circumstances of bankruptcy, debt collections, and looming threat of asset repossession. John paid for our sessions in cash, a rarity in these times of bank transfers and credit cards. Retrieving a bundle of cash from his pocket, John would reel off notes haphazardly, splaying them on the sideboard as he left the session. He remains the only patient who has ever encouraged me to 'keep the change'.

What was he communicating to me by paying in cash, insisting I keep the change? Was I another woman to be kept, or one that needed to be cared for as his mother had needed from him? Was this a way to impress me? A way to keep me in his life as he had tried to do with his estranged wife? Perhaps wealth was a marker of success to John, an effort to match his father's financial achievements. Money had allowed John to change his mother's life; he had told me of the feeling of pride when he was able to move his mother from the council flat into a stand-alone house in an affluent suburb. The recent bankruptcy – and whatever business activities surrounded it, legal or otherwise – had challenged his notion of success, and challenged his ability to help others. Bankruptcy seemed reminiscent of his father leaving, with John being left destitute in both instances. John had become adept at being the responsible one, skilled at rescuing people. He used money as a mechanism to repair and recover, forging his way through the significant difficulties he had encountered.

In later sessions, we spoke more about John's family, focusing on the eventual reconciliation with his father and introduction to the 'new family'. John's half-siblings had enjoyed a remarkably different upbringing from John and his brothers. The lifestyle benefits that came with their father's improved financial circumstances were one obvious factor. The other and more pertinent element was the care his father showed for John's half-siblings. He was present and engaged, attentive to their needs. The doting father role seemed so removed from the man who left his 'first family', the man who did not look back at his four young sons as they watched him walk away. The emotional deprivation – that is, the lack of attention and care towards the children's emotional needs – experienced by John and his siblings was left undiscussed with their father.

"He was a turncoat," John exclaimed, using an expression I had not heard in years. John spoke of resentment for his half-siblings, feeling they were afforded opportunities at the expense of John and his brothers.

John maintained a relationship with his father and half-siblings. "I wanted to remind them of who I was, that he couldn't just leave like that. I wouldn't let him forget us."

"Those feelings are absolutely valid, John. You experienced the way you and your brothers were living, your mum fending for you all. It seems that your half-siblings lived in another world. The contrast between your council flat and their nice place by the seaside. I wonder what that was like for you?"

"I always felt like the poor cousin at any family event. We just knew we were different. He'd given up on us, everyone knew that."

The shame was still raw. John glanced down, unable to maintain eye contact in that moment. The shame at being the forgotten family, the deserted family, the family left to eat tinned beans on toast.

Shame had peppered John's life. Shame at being abandoned by his father, of not being able to provide a meal for his brothers on the night their father left. Shame at living in poverty, at being thrice divorced, at again finding himself in financial dire straits. The experience of shame is deep-seated, a core emotion located in the subcortical region of the brain. It is often unspoken and implicit; it is felt as distress, disconnection, or discomfort, but often the impetus or cause of the feeling is not able to be identified or articulated.

John was now proving himself to be anything but the poor cousin. His flash car and rolls of cash represented an overt sign of his new place in the world. I reflected this to John; he had established himself in a world in which the odds were stacked against him. These outward markers of success seemed to do little to mitigate John's emotional distress.

"It's all for nought though, isn't it?" he answered quickly, his voice cracking.

John's pining conveyed a sense of desperation. "It's just *stuff*. I don't have anyone. They're all gone. Everyone has left. *Capisce?!*"

Abandonment. John was feeling not only the sting of his recent marital separation, but also many re-opened wounds: his parents' divorce, his father leaving, the love and attention deserved by him given instead to his half-siblings. Adverse childhood experiences are never far from our minds; feelings of distress are swiftly triggered by events we experience later in life that are in some way reminiscent of earlier trauma.

I asked John about his half-siblings; it seemed they were close at one stage, but that had given way to a new kind of acrimony and estrangement in recent years.

"I was always jealous of them. They went to proper schools, got good jobs. Everything presented on a silver platter. They couldn't fail in life. Sometimes, I just wished they would know how we felt. I wanted them to hit some barriers, know the feeling of being left behind."

"You thought some of your hurt would heal if they also experienced pain?"

John nodded in agreement.

"We often look to the people who have hurt us to heal us. We think the solution is for others to feel what we have felt. But, in truth, the people who hurt us won't be those that heal us."

A long pause between us. I let the silence extend, sensing John had more to say. John was staring at his hands. Rough hands with grease stains and chipped fingernails, the top of one finger missing. The hands of a person who had experienced hard work in his years. I imagined the difference between John's hands and those of his half-siblings, picturing smooth skin and manicured nails. My mind drifted; images of those manicured hands holding champagne flutes and toasting good fortune, while John sat in the front bar of a dingy pub, trading war stories and placing bets.

I prompted John after a few more minutes. "John, what's going through your mind at the moment?" I asked softly, careful to capture his attention by preceding my question with his name.

"That you should be careful what you wish for," John replied quickly and with intent. This seemed a statement over which he had reflected and ruminated. Our eyes met. I noticed his were red, his cheeks stained with tears. He quickly returned his gaze to his hands, continuing to study the well-worn creases as if they were new to him.

"Tell me more, John . . . " John was ready to speak, to let it all out. And out it flowed.

"What really broke me," he began, pausing as his voice broke, "was everything with Simone. It broke us all. The whole family was shattered. We've never recovered. It was twenty years ago. It feels like yesterday."

I paused for a moment, taking in the information. Images of champagne and beer quickly evacuated my mind.

Simone. *Simone.* Twenty years ago. I counted back the years in my mind. Yes, it had been twenty years. The picture of a beautiful young woman sprung into my mind, followed by a shudder of realisation that she would forever be 19 years old. Simone had been dead for twenty years. Could we be thinking of the same Simone? Could it be? Surely not.

I was facing a professional dilemma. Such considerations abound in therapy. This was not the first time I had experienced a professional or ethical issue, and it would certainly not be the last. But this felt different. Maybe it was the intensity of the therapy with John, our strong therapeutic rapport, compounded by the magnitude of this event in his life. This triggered my own thoughts, leading me to feeling transported back in time, finding myself thinking about the events of twenty years ago.

My usual strategies when facing decisions with potential ethical ramifications include taking time to sit on a decision, seeking supervision, and talking to colleagues. Training dictates that my usual practice is to record the decision and all steps towards it. But in that moment, I made a split-second decision. I remembered the wisdom of Carl Jung: "know all the theories, master all the techniques, but as you touch a human soul be just another human soul." I was a human with another human sitting in front of me. For all its technicalities and modalities, sometimes therapy is as simple (and complicated) as that.

"I know Simone," I blurted out the words, not quite recognising my own voice.

John stared back at me, mouth agape and eyes widened.

"I *knew* Simone," I added, quickly correcting my confusion of past and present tense. "We were at university together. We studied together, before . . . "

My voice drifted off. I was saying too much. I wanted to sweep up my words, put them back where they had been for twenty years. But it was too late, the information was known, the cat was out of the bag, and the relationship between John and me would never be the same.

I remembered Simone. Not many could forget her. A tall girl with long golden hair. I was envious of her beauty and confidence. I felt like an ugly duckling in her presence. She seemed aware of her stature, intelligence, the sway she held over men and women alike. These characteristics that can so often lead to jealousy were buffered by Simone's even temperament and kind nature. She seemed to exist in the world with an ease far beyond her years.

Simone and I sat together in our first-year psychology lecture. The lecturer was expounding about relationships, telling us that most humans have sex in the dark, and that humans are the only species who will intentionally seek a dark space to engage in sexual intercourse. Giggling erupted throughout the auditorium; a bunch of adolescents apparently coy at the mention of sex. Simone turned to me, her hair swishing effortlessly with the movement of her head. Her light-hearted laughter contrasted with the stupendous giggling of our classmates.

"Seriously, who would have sex in the dark? What a waste!" she whispered to me as the lecturer attempted to return some sense of order among the rowdy students. I nodded nervously in agreement, pretending to be as worldly and experienced as Simone seemed to assume of me.

I thought of the comment at her funeral two months later.

What a waste.

The scene ticked over and over in my mind. Simone's laugh, her golden hair, her broad smile, her poise, her *joie de vivre*. It seemed impossible to reconcile that the bright and bubbly young woman was lying in the casket at the front of the church.

Lying in darkness. What a waste.

Mourners filed in, quickly filling the pews. A surplus of people hovered at the back of the church. Her parents and siblings distraught, friends sobbing, a group united in grief for the loss of Simone. Pop music and uplifting eulogies designed to encourage mourners to celebrate rather than mourn Simone's life did little to lift the heavy shadow of the sombre mood.

Adults (did I not yet consider myself an adult?) at the funeral and wake commented on the *waste* of a young life, the *waste* of opportunity, the *waste* of it all.

What a waste.

The solemn state extended to our drive home. A small group of university friends, seemingly aged overnight by the death of our friend. The disbelief that we were here and Simone was not. For most of us this was our first exposure to the vulnerability and impermanence of human life. Thus far our time together as a cohort of young students had been marked by events that now seemed wildly petty and embarrassingly insignificant – overdue assignments, beastly hangovers, love triangles, light-hearted arguments over whether our 6 pm viewing should be *The Simpsons* or the nightly news.

I considered sharing with my fellow passengers the anecdote from our psychology lecture. I wanted to console them. Simone had a short life, but a good life. She was confident. She even enjoyed having sex with the lights on! It sounded absurd as I repeated the sentence in my head. I kept it to myself, realising this titbit of information could never be conveyed in a way that captured the spirit of the moment shared between Simone and me.

Unbeknownst to me, John was among the mourners at the funeral. We couldn't have guessed that our lives would intersect in a therapy room some two decades later. John asked me for my recollections of Simone. She was a beautiful young woman, I told him. Kind and caring, well-respected. I had no doubt she would have excelled in any field of work or study, I continued. Her life, I added as I reached for a glass of water to calm the quiver of my voice, was too short.

What a waste, I thought silently.

So often in therapy I have heard stories of loss, heartbreak, despair. I have always listened intently and with a genuine sense of empathy. But never before had I known such insight into a patient's experience. In that moment I truly understood the notion of empathy being not something that is given but rather something that is experienced by the recipient.

"I *knew* I chose you for a reason! I knew it!" John reiterated, slapping his hand on his knee as a smile crept across his face.

The coincidence was meaningful to John. It was meaningful to us both. I again recalled Jung, a contemporary of Sigmund Freud and a revered psychoanalyst and theorist in his own right, and thought how he might look at the story of John as exemplary of synchronicity. Jung posited that synchronicity is a meaningful coincidence, an event on the outside that speaks to something on the inside, an external event that has significant internal meaning. This is distinct from a random occurrence. An example of this may be thinking of an acquaintance whom you have not seen for many years, then bumping into that same person at the supermarket. You would likely exclaim how uncanny it was to see them, having just thought of that person after a long absence. Life is full of synchronous moments, if only we allow ourselves to be open to the experiences.

The connection between Simone and me, however tenuous, was important to helping John. Any kind of connection, any flicker of memory of Simone so powerful that it was perceived to be some kind of fateful intervention. John had tried to make sense of his experience of Simone's death for so many years; I imagined thoughts and feelings whirling around his mind like an infinite cycle of laundry in a washing machine.

John filled in some gaps around Simone's life. I was saddened to hear of the death of Simone's mother a few years after her daughter. The cumulative grief had overwhelmed Simone's father. I thought of the stoic man at his daughter's funeral, of the cruel nature of a world in which a person could lose both his daughter and wife in quick succession. It was heartening to hear of the lives of Simone's siblings – pursuing study, establishing careers, and starting families of their own.

The trials and tribulations of a family, summarised in a few minutes. Our brief existence and minuscule place in the vast universe, seemingly a paradox with the intensity of grief that can come from the loss of just one person.

Simone's father was John's younger half-sibling, making Simone John's niece. The pieces were falling into place. The family tree I was sketching in my mind suddenly took shape and gained meaning. The significance of the acrimonious relationship between John and his younger half-sibling became apparent; John resented Simone's father and spent a great deal of his life experiencing feelings of hatred and envy towards him. John perceived their early life to be picture-perfect, a life that John felt had been stripped away with his father's departure, handed instead to Simone's father and his siblings.

"I wished for something bad to happen to them. And. It. Did."

It was a *mea culpa*. A declaration years in the making. Here was John, putting words to a lifetime of pain and guilt. In doing this, John was proclaiming his toxicity: he was a toxic person whom people abandoned – his father, and subsequently three wives. Difficult business dealings and bankruptcy also gave a sense of toxicity, a feeling that he also spoiled professional as well as personal situations. John's image of himself was dominated by these parts; he was unable to view his whole self without it being contaminated by these parts he viewed as less desirable.

Therapists hear many 'confessions'. More admissions of infidelity than I can count on both hands. Pregnancies terminated without the knowledge of a partner or parent. Others wishing they had never become parents. Cheating on high school exams. Reading others' text messages and snooping on emails. Opening another person's mail and finding more information than bargained for. Secluding assets and cash from a partner or family member, not trusting their intentions.

I remind myself to never take this privilege for granted. It is no easy feat for patients to speak aloud shameful secrets, to share innermost thoughts, to express concerns that have kept them awake at night, to speak that which has been captive in their minds. Such declarations are sometimes followed with the patient stating they will understand if I no longer want to work with them; their 'crimes' are so heinous that they expect rejection (and have most likely experienced rejection from others in whom they may have confided). One person told me they understood that I would judge them for their choices around terminating a pregnancy. The pained expression on their face conveyed their shame. I told them my honest thoughts – that they were giving themself a hard enough time, there was no need for further degradation from me. We worked together for years; further revelations of what they considered shameful secrets revealed as our therapeutic rapport grew and the trust between us was further fostered.

John had been carrying this thought for twenty years. In his mind, it was a simple equation – he wished ill upon his father's children, and now one of them had experienced the death of their child. Arguably, there is no greater pain that can be endured than parents' loss of a child. I recalled an elderly patient's comments on the death of his young granddaughter, reflecting on his son: "I will forgive him almost anything, as he has experienced the immeasurable anguish of losing a child."

John had been tortured by these thoughts. He had tortured himself with the thoughts. We unpacked these further, working on the subconscious notion of his toxicity and deservedness of experiencing his father leaving and the dissolution of three marriages. He knew logically that his thoughts did not cause Simone's death, but the guilt he felt for bringing his toxicity into the lives of others was being projected onto Simone's death. This magical thinking seemed to fall short of a delusion; John's thoughts about

Simone were rigid but not impenetrable. Magical thinking, typified by loose connections between thoughts, offers a subverted way to make sense of odd life events and strange happenings. It is a common thinking pattern for trauma survivors and those experiencing post-traumatic stress disorder (PTSD).

"A thought is not a fact, John," I said, my tone firm and direct as I introduced a cognitive-behavioural therapy principle of challenging unhelpful thoughts. "Don't believe everything you think. I could think the couch you're sitting on is red, but it doesn't change the fact that it's actually blue."

John gave a wry smile. Taking the focus away from Simone and her death had enacted some kind of change, some kind of switch that opened a new therapeutic path to be explored. John's feelings of toxicity and guilt were core beliefs, present long before Simone's death but arguably reinforced by it. Her death provided a catalyst and opportunity for these to be discussed, the synchronicity derived from our shared connection with Simone lending itself to a unique rapport.

I continued, encouraged by John's enthusiastic smile and bright eyes.

"Of *course* you were resentful! Life was tough. Your dad left, your mum was forced to fend for herself – and *four* kids. You, being the eldest, could see what might have been, how your life would have been different if your father had channelled his energy into your family. Instead, he got a 'new family'. A glamorous life on the coast in contrast to your life in the council flat. Who wouldn't be resentful of that?! I sure as hell would be!"

I momentarily wondered if I had gone too far with my summary of John's experience. Reflecting information back to patients in such a way can sometimes be distressing, but John instead seemed energised.

"I made good though, Bianca! I made good! I worked and worked, got Mum out of the council flat! You seen my car?"

A palpable sense of pride. A glimmer of bravado, a hint of the swagger fitting of a person driving a sports car. I told John I had seen his car and wouldn't mind a similar one, sharing that it was also an object of admiration among my colleagues.

"You sure did make good, John," I continued with genuine enthusiasm. "And that is your doing. You have everything to be proud of. But Simone's death was *not* your doing."

We sat in silence for a few moments.

John could be labelled as experiencing complex grief. Difficult relationships with a person during their life usually predict complexities in mourning, with grief that does not typically resolve within an unexpected time frame or follow the trajectory typical of that experienced by most individuals following a death. His thoughts about causing Simone's death by wishing harm to her father and his family could be considered magical thinking at best, delusional at worst. I didn't consider any of these things. My copy of the DSM-V (the so-called 'diagnostic bible') stayed unopened on the shelf. Instead, I saw a man trapped by his own thoughts, a prisoner of his own experiences, a product of some particularly nasty twists and turns in this strange journey we call life. John didn't need a diagnosis, he needed understanding and care.

John was a human, talking to another human, expressing his fragility, seeking connection, hoping for something to shift this terminal state. It is, as Irvin Yalom so eloquently reminds us, the relationship that heals. John needed permission to think a different way, to loosen the shackles of toxicity, to confront the guilt that had infiltrated his life for two decades.

"John, you did nothing wrong. There is no way that you contributed to or caused Simone's death." I leaned forward, sustaining eye contact and speaking clearly. "Forgive yourself, John. Forgive yourself."

I felt a connection with John as I said the words. I was telling him to forgive himself, but the words also resonated with me in an unexpected way. In that moment, I realised I too had felt a sense of guilt around Simone's death. My admiration of her beauty and confidence had been tinged with envy, just as John had felt towards Simone's father. The origins of our envy differed; his underpinned by a toxicity in wishing ill-harm, mine driven by an immature veneration. I felt a sense of remorse for living a life that was already twice as long as hers, for having experiences and opportunities she would never enjoy.

John stood up from the couch, glanced at the clock, telling me it was time for him to go. He left the usual bundle of cash on the sideboard. I listened as the door to the clinic closed, the engine of the sports car revved, and the tyres skidded along the gravel driveway.

I wasn't sure I would see John again. But he attended our next session, and dozens more after that. I wondered if this was his way of confronting his deep-seated feelings of toxicity; he would not allow our therapeutic relationship to be ruined, despite the difficult and confronting ground we had covered. I had not abandoned him, and he was not abandoning me.

We never again spoke of Simone. That chapter, it seemed, was closed.

FURTHER READING

Codrington, R. (2017). Trauma, Dissociation, and Chronic Shame – Reflections for Couple and Family Practice: An Interview with Kathy Steele. *Australian and New Zealand Journal of Family Therapy*, *38*(4), 669–679. https://doi.org/10.1002/anzf.1275

Cook, D. R. (1991). Shame, attachment, and addictions: Implications for family therapists. *Contemporary Family Therapy*, *13*(5), 405–419. https://doi.org/10.1007/BF00890495

Denny, B. (2023, 6 November). How shame influences the decisions we make, and compounds the harm we do to others. *ABC Religion & Ethics*. https://www.abc.net.au/religion/shame-regret-and-the-reasons-for-the-decisions-we-make/103070984

Diagnostic and statistical manual of mental disorders: DSM-5 (5th ed. Special ed.). (2017). CBS Publishers & Distributors, Pvt. Ltd.

Eubanks, C. F. (2022). Rupture Repair. *Cognitive and Behavioral Practice*, *29*(3), 554–559. https://doi.org/10.1016/j.cbpra.2022.02.012

Jung, C. G. (1995). *Synchronicity: An acausal connecting principle* (repr). ARK Paperbacks.

Mullainathan, S., & Shafir, E. (2014). *Scarcity: The true cost of not having enough*. Penguin Books.

Riker, J. H. (2024). *Kohut's self psychology for a fractured world: New ways of understanding the self and human community*. Routledge.

Rogers, C. R. (2004). *On becoming a person: A therapist's view of psychotherapy*. Constable.

Schwartz, R. C. (2021). *No bad parts: Healing trauma and restoring wholeness*. Vermilion.

Winnicott, D. W. (with Winnicott, C., Shepherd, R., & Davis, M.). (2014). *Home is where we start from: Essays by a psychoanalyst*. W.W. Norton & Company.

Wolynn, M. (2017). *It didn't start with you: How inherited family trauma shapes who we are and how to end the cycle*. Penguin Books.

Yalom, I. D. (2013). *Love's executioner and other tales of psychotherapy* (new ed.). Penguin Books.

Young, J. E. (with Klosko, J. S., & Beck, A. T.). (1994). *Reinventing your life: The breakthrough program to end negative behavior . . . and feel great again*. Penguin Publishing Group.

2

WASH, RINSE, REPEAT

History repeats itself, but in such cunning disguise that we never detect the resemblance until the damage is done.

Sydney J. Harris

I had arrived at work early, feeling a little smug after beating the morning traffic and reaching work earlier than a notoriously eager colleague. I wanted to get a head-start on what was looking to be a busy day. In that moment, I was comfortable, acting as close to my non-professional self as I ever would at work; alone at the consulting rooms, with no patients and other clinicians yet to arrive. A new patient, Luke, was scheduled for my first appointment.

Balancing a hot cup of tea in one hand and a pile of papers in the other, I deftly kicked the consulting room door closed behind me.

I shrieked as I turned around, feeling the sting of boiling hot water as it splashed on my leg. A man was sitting on the couch.

"I'm so sorry! Sorry, sorry, *sorry!*" He quickly leapt up, taking the papers out of my hand.

Tall and lanky with floppy hair and kind brown eyes, the sight of him was more of a surprise than a threat.

"I wasn't sure where I was meant to wait! So, I just sat in here! Nice room, by the way," he added, glancing around at its high ceilings, pointing towards the large windows through which the morning sunlight was beginning to creep.

"You gave me a fright!" I laughed, as I composed myself. "Luke, I assume?"

Bypassing the waiting room, I later thought, was the first indication of an important characteristic of Luke's personality – his tendency to set himself apart from others. He marked himself as different. Normal rules did not apply to him. He was not just another patient. Luke was special, and deserved special treatment.

In subsequent sessions, Luke continued to bypass the waiting room. He would let himself into my consulting room, where I would find him browsing through a book from my bookshelf, inspecting artwork on the wall, and – one time – adjusting the thermostat.

DOI: 10.4324/9781003621645-3

I never saw Luke enter the building. Nor did I hear him. This was odd; Nepalese-style chimes hanging from the door handle invariably alerted us to the arrival of patients.

Luke shirked my requests for him to sit in the waiting room until called. He laughed in response, asking why he would wait "out there" when he could sit comfortably in this room. In retrospect, this initial boundary crossing and my reluctance to more strongly enforce it marked the beginning of a challenging power dynamic in our therapeutic relationship.

Forty-five-year-old Luke was experiencing intense distress following the recent break-down of his relationship with Rebecca. The three-year on-off relationship was typified by an ongoing conflict, one not uncommon among couples: Rebecca, a decade younger than Luke, was eager to marry and start a family, contrasting sharply with Luke's reluctance to commit to her and the idea of having children.

The precarious balance between adventure and safety is an integral and ongoing struggle of the human psyche. We crave security, yet often find ourselves engaging in behaviour counterintuitive to obtaining and maintaining this. For many, safety and security are assumed to take the form of a monogamous long-term relationship.

But what happens when we get what we want? And why do so many people seemingly fall out of love with the idea of this – and their partner and the life they envisioned together – as quickly as they fall into it?

Luke spoke at length about his relationship with Rebecca. In fact, Rebecca was all we spoke of for several sessions. I wondered if this was an indication of limerence (an all-consuming infatuation or obsession with a romantic interest). I asked Luke how much time he spent thinking of or talking about Rebecca; his response of "every waking moment" came as little surprise. While seemingly obsessed with her and the end of their relationship, Luke did not seem to present any danger to Rebecca. He was not stalking Rebecca, nor did it seem the contact was unwanted, objected to, or perceived by Rebecca to be threatening. Their relationship seemed a strange type of mutual obsession, a co-dependence of sorts.

The two had been in an on-again-off-again relationship for several years. Breaks in the relationship were usually initiated by Luke. Somewhat paradoxically this occurred when he felt especially fond of Rebecca or the two had spent an extended period of time together. He warned her about getting too close to him, often repeating his mantra of never wanting marriage or children. Rebecca was wasting her time with him, Luke would remind her, willing her to find someone who shared her dreams of domesticity and white picket fences.

During our early sessions, Luke had demonstrated strong conviction in his opposition to marriage and children. He boasted about enjoying his bachelor status and bragged about the freedom that came with it. Luke enjoyed travel, often making last-minute plans and taking advantage of flight and accommodation specials. He didn't particularly relish the company of small children, comfortable in the 'Fun Uncle' role but happily handing children back to their parents at the first hint of a dirty nappy or toddler tantrum. He had concerns about balancing the care needs of his elderly mother with the inevitable obligations his own children would bring. Luke was clear: he didn't want to be tied down.

Rebecca's dominance of our sessions was an apt reflection of her dominance in Luke's thoughts. Only when prompted would Luke provide even scant history of his family background. He was similarly reluctant to speak about his work as a teacher, denying it was central to any of his current concerns. This seemed unusual. I have worked with many teachers; vocation is invariably central to their identity and work is often intertwined with the reason for engaging in therapy. As is true of many professions, teachers usually need little prompting to discuss work. Luke seemed quite the opposite to the characteristics usual to teachers – conscientiousness, respectfulness, and, for some, perfectionism.

"I gotta come clean with you, Doc," Luke began as soon as I entered the room for our eighth session. As had become customary, Luke had let himself into the consulting room. He was seated on the couch, impatience indicated by rapid tapping of his feet. He continued to greet me as 'Doc', one of very few patients who did not adhere to my preference for use of my first name over any professional title.

I walked in with my usual cup of tea. Having a hot drink in session was not a habit for me, but became standard during sessions with Luke. Perhaps my response to him breaking the rules was to bend a habit of my own. In retrospect, this seemed another indication of my accommodation of his behaviour, another small but significant sign of the dynamic developing within our therapeutic relationship.

"My name is not Luke. And I am not a teacher."

Conscious of my surprised facial expression, I raised my ubiquitous cup of tea, removing the tea bag and placing it on a tissue on the table between us. I watched Luke's eyes watch the teabag, its sepia tone quickly spreading across the tissue. I cradled the mug in my hands, taking a long sip of tea before regaining eye contact with him.

"But I swear everything else is true! *Everything!*" Luke was staring at me, a look of pleading on his face.

"Whew." I surprised myself with the casual response.

Whew is not likely a response you would read in a counselling textbook. Nor is it likely one I would make with many patients. In a training workshop or role play with a colleague, I would likely have responded with an acknowledgement of the statement, following an expression of gratitude for the patient sharing such difficult information. As a trainee I would have been sheepish about sharing that part of the session with my supervisor. But in some ways being a trainee therapist is akin to learning to drive; techniques and general rules are learned while training, then therapists increasingly develop their own style. Therapy becomes a dynamic interaction, guided by knowledge, intuition, common sense, and experience.

My surprise was genuine, as was my expression of *whew*. I had thought a few things were remiss in Luke's recollection of events, but that in and of itself was not unusual. People experiencing psychological distress often emphasise or minimise events in keeping with their own narrative.

Most patients take a while to warm up to therapy, especially those new to the process. Few patients immediately disclose their true reason for attending. Many test the waters with the extent and type of information, attempting to ascertain whether this therapist can be trusted with their deepest thoughts and long-held secrets. In this way, the development of a therapeutic relationship is not unlike any other relationship; over time, layers of modesty give way to comfort and honesty.

We had delved into deep and dark aspects of his life, but an assumed name gave 'Luke' anonymity, distance, and – perhaps most pertinently – an opportunity to leave therapy without any way for his absence to be queried or followed up.

This strategy of having an exit plan seemed a reflection of Luke's avoidant attachment style. This was playing out in our therapeutic relationship, just as it likely did in other relationships in his life. The therapy room, as revered psychotherapist Irvin Yalom suggests, is a microcosm of the patient's broader world; happenings in the therapy room mirror the patient's external world, and, perhaps most importantly, can impact change in the patient's external world.

I knew it was important to hold space for Luke. I did this by focusing on the revelation as an implicit invitation to learn more about him, rather than perceiving the withholding of information as a betrayal.

"It sounds like we have a lot to catch up on. Where shall we start?"

Daniel, as I came to know him, came and went from therapy. He preferred not to set regular session times, often requesting last-minute appointments via text message or email. More than once I forfeited a lunch break to accommodate an appointment request. I felt somehow compelled to meet his demands, thus allowing another incremental step down the slippery slope of lax boundaries and informality that had come to typify our therapeutic relationship. I submitted to Daniel's entitlement and the power dynamic dictated by his egotism.

Attendance at a flurry of session – up to three per week – was bookended by absences of weeks or months. He attributed this to an unpredictable work schedule. Over time, however, I came to view this pattern of engagement in therapy as reflective of his relationship with Rebecca: hot then cold, in then out, enthusiastic then withdrawn.

A self-proclaimed 'epiphany' had prompted Daniel's most recent re-engagement in therapy. During yet another break in his relationship with Rebecca, Daniel had realised that he was ready for marriage and children. Nothing had been clearer in his life, Daniel reported. He couldn't believe he had been so remiss for so many years. Daniel likened the realisation to seeing an optical illusion; once he had seen the truth and the way forward, it could not be unseen.

Daniel and Rebecca had remained in contact while 'on a break' from their relationship. Both were back on the dating scene. Daniel laughed as he recalled trading light-hearted stories with her about lame first dates and dead-end chats on online dating apps.

Daniel invited Rebecca to dinner. He summoned the courage to express his regret for his past indecision. He apologised for hurting her. He understood why her friends and family had likely told her to run a mile from him. Daniel declared to Rebecca that he was now ready to fully commit to a life together. There was no time to waste. Yes, he wanted children! Yes, he wanted children with her! Yes, *yes*, YES! Let's get started, he joked.

I was perched on the edge of my chair, listening to Daniel's animated recall of the dinner date. Daniel was quite the raconteur. And he knew it. Hands flailing and eyes widening, voice peaking to a crescendo to add emphasis, dipping to a diminuendo to build tension. I felt enthused by his energy, hanging on his every word. I was silently cheering for Daniel, willing a happy ending. I supressed a niggling yet obvious thought – that good news was unlikely to precede Daniel scheduling a therapy session.

Daniel's voice lowered. A deep sigh, marking a change of tone and drop in energy. He had fidgeted during the dinner, he recalled, feeling the outline of a jewellery box in the pocket of his jacket. He had planned to propose to Rebecca.

My heart sank a little. I leaned back into my chair, readying myself for the inevitable turn of the story.

Rebecca raised her hand, Daniel recalled, urging him to stop as he laughed at his own joke about making a start on making a family.

Daniel shook his head, a retrospective grimace at his own corny gag. He inhaled deeply and raised his head, shrugging his shoulders as if to shake himself back into the present moment.

Her manner was different, he mused. They would usually be in bed together by this stage of a reconciliation dinner, he joked. She seemed thoroughly unimpressed, impatient even. So foreign was this nonchalant response from Rebecca that he wondered what he had done to deserve this frosty reception.

Rebecca replied in the most unexpected of ways. She had recently started dating someone. It had quickly become serious. He had met her parents, been endorsed by her friends. Marriage and children had already been discussed. She was committed to this new relationship. He was committed to this new relationship. They were committed to this new relationship. Together, they were committed. Daniel's efforts were too little, too late. Sorry, she offered. That ship has sailed.

Rebecca left before the main meal was served. Daniel was left staring at her half-glass of wine and an untouched piece of buttered bread. Stunned, he stumbled out of the restaurant, reminded of the bill only when a waiter confronted him in the car park.

"'That ship has sailed!' Can you believe she said that to me? As if I'm *nothing* to her. Apparently those three years meant *absolutely nothing* to her."

I said very little during the session. Daniel seemed skittish and agitated, jumping around the chronology of the events of dinner. He recalled the details over and over, increasingly incredulous at its ending. He was annoyed at Rebecca's use of the naval cliché, perceiving this dismissal of their relationship to be unceremonious and disrespectful.

"I'm back on the dating apps. Two can play at this game!"

"What game is that, Daniel?" It was as close as I came to any type of challenging statement.

"I'm as good as she was ever going to get. I'll show her what she's missing. I've got a date tonight," he continued, without any acknowledgement of my query.

The session morphed from a dialogue to monologue. He showed no interest in my thoughts and no inclination towards any of his being discussed or contested. Daniel's response was narcissistic; he had the floor and I was simply his audience.

Daniel smiled wryly, retrieving his phone and swiping to a photo of a woman who bore a striking resemblance to Rebecca.

"I know what you're thinking," Daniel started. "Yes, I have a type." He held up both his hands and scrunched his face, as if pre-emptively surrendering to the judgement he expected from me.

I thought this rapid return to dating and his adoption of a triumphant position may be indicative of an unconscious attempt by Daniel to deny the distress arising from Rebecca's rejection. Daniel could not tolerate the distress and difficult feelings subsequent to the dinner with Rebecca. Instead, he rebounded onto the dating scene with lightning speed. This was an attempt to prove, both to himself and others, his attractiveness and desirability.

"I'll come back tomorrow. What time have you got? Can you squeeze me in? Come on, Doc . . . you know I need to see you."

I reflected on the work with Daniel thus far. The ongoing sporadic and disjointed nature of sessions added to my thinking about his attachment style. Other relationships in his life were also sporadic and disjointed. I began to wonder if the relationship with his caregivers during the early years of his life reflected a similar pattern. In some way, had that time in his life set him up for these transactional and disorganised relationships? It seemed Daniel was re-enacting the pattern of relationships best known to him.

"Well, she wasn't Rebecca," Daniel offered when I asked how his date had been. "The sex was fine," he shrugged. He had no intention of seeing the woman again. Sexual gratification provided an anaesthesia for Daniel's distress. This relief, however, was short-lived.

"I just can't stop thinking about Rebecca. I've made the biggest mistake of my life."

"I wonder if there's any other times in your life you've felt like this? Previous girlfriends, relationships, friendships that have ended . . .?"

This was an attempt to re-direct the focus from Rebecca. An effort to look more broadly across Daniel's life to test the idea that his experiences with Rebecca were not an anomaly, but rather a reflection of some sort of repetition compulsion. I suspected that Daniel may be unconsciously compelled to repeat embedded behaviour and patterns within relationships.

"Yeah, I suppose. Once in my twenties. My girlfriend of the time, Paula. Gee, she was good-looking. Long legs, dark hair . . ." Daniel's voice drifted off, lost in the dreamy recollection of Paula.

"She wanted to settle down. I just wasn't ready. I tried to get her back a few years later, but she had already moved on. Ha, I thought that was the most heartbroken I would ever be in my life! But this . . ." Daniel shook his head.

"You tried to 'get her back?'" I queried, mirroring his own language.

"Yeah. We had been exchanging messages, keeping up with each other's lives. Paula stayed beautiful. She got more beautiful as she aged, if that's even possible! She had moved to Brisbane. I said I would move up there. A fresh start for both of us. I was ready to go, all packed up, but Paula pulled the pin. She told me not to come."

"What was that like for you?"

"I was heartbroken. Devastated. I had it all planned out. I was ready for it, ready for her, ready to settle down."

"Seems history has repeated itself . . .?" I offered.

"S'pose it has. Yeah, it has."

The focus was off Rebecca, onto Daniel's experiences over time. There was a sense of momentum and direction in the session. Finally, we were getting somewhere.

"And with anyone else? Have you experienced this with anyone else?"

"Sometimes with my mates. They ask me to do something and then cut me out of the plans when I don't answer quick enough. I tell them I can't just say 'yes' straight away because of my work schedule. And then they go ahead without me. It happened with a football game a few weeks ago. I would have liked to go. Turned out to be a great game, winning kick after the siren. And they all went to Bali without me. That was tough. If I was on social media I sure as hell wouldn't have checked it during that week!"

Daniel often referred to his absence from social media. He was suspicious of the way such sites collected and used data. But Daniel's absence from these channels also meant he was omitted from social opportunities and missed updates about friends' lives, often resulting in feelings of being ignored or out of the loop.

The picture of Daniel's attachment style and his experience of relationships was becoming clearer. Daniel had shied away from commitment throughout his life, only to have opportunities expire before he had felt ready to embrace them. Time and time again, he had rejected and then been rejected. This was an ongoing pattern with friends and also notable within two significant romantic relationships. Moreover, this was not dissimilar to the pattern of our sessions. Daniel would reject my offer of scheduling sessions in advance, then respond with a terse *'I guess I'll just have to make do'* text message if I was not able to meet his demand for an appointment at short notice.

Daniel was unconsciously setting up situations in which he may experience rejection. This self-sabotage seemed to play out in several aspects of his life. His epiphany regarding commitment to Rebecca after years of indecision could be seen as an ultimate act of self-sabotage. He would suffer and be special in his suffering.

"I wonder if that's a kind of self-sabotage, Daniel? Rejecting an opportunity, then feeling rejected and disappointed when that opportunity is no longer available to you." I paused, wanting a chance for the statement to sink in. "I notice it with our sessions, too," I continued. "You decline my offer of a regular session time, then it seems you are a bit pissed off when I'm not always able to accommodate your request for a last-minute appointment. It's as if you are reluctant to commit, then become upset when I cannot reciprocate when you decide you are ready to commit to sessions."

"Are you saying that I treat you the same as my girlfriends? Look, Doc, you're an attractive woman and all, I would definitely swipe right, but . . ." Daniel shot me a smile and a wink.

"Thanks, Daniel." I smiled at his light-hearted attempt at deflection.

I pushed on. "There's a pattern in your relationships. Whether that's with me, your work as an on-call employee, friendships, or romantic relationships. I know this whole thing with Rebecca has been devastating. And there's a few things that have contributed to that. The way all these events, this repeated pattern of behaviour, the way these relationships have ended. . . how much has all this taken its toll on you . . .?"

Daniel was quiet. We sat in silence for a minute or so.

"Daniel, it seems there is an ongoing internal conflict. You long for attachment, but the implications of commitment terrify you. So, you sabotage situations which offer a glimpse of that security and commitment."

"I bring this on myself."

It was a statement, not a question. A sign of realisation, or perhaps resignation. Daniel had identified that he was punishing himself. But of what did he unconsciously believe he was guilty?

"Not consciously," I continued. "When patterns are familiar, we end up falling into them time and time again. Like a familiar road that you've driven down a hundred times. You don't even think about taking a different road, even though that route might be a better option. A kind of mindlessness. Humans are creatures of habit. We are all creatures of habit."

More silence.

Daniel was quiet, contemplative. After a few minutes, I asked what was going through his mind. Could he share his thoughts with me?

"It makes sense. But, shit . . . I'm a bloody mess. I've screwed it all up."

I asked Daniel who he may be able to look to for support and company during this time.

"I've worn out my welcome with all my mates. Their wives are getting shirty about the heartbroken loser crashing on the couch. Uncle Daniel ain't much fun around the kids at the moment."

"How about your Mum?"

"No, no, no, no, *no*. She wouldn't have that. She would tell me to pull up my socks and get on with it. Don't cry over spilt milk. I don't need to be reminded that I've made a big mistake. *Mistakes*. Big mistakes."

"Your Mum would press that onto you?"

Daniel had spoken of a strong relationship with his mother. He had an enduring respect for her. She was a permanent, if slightly distant, figure in an otherwise unstable childhood. The family enjoyed financial privilege, but severe emotional deprivation as a consequence of his father's verbal and physical abuse of Daniel's mother and his siblings.

Daniel often commended his mother's achievement of raising a family in adverse circumstances. However, he also acknowledged that her pragmatism and capacity for dealing with difficult situations came at the expense of maternal warmth. Daniel had very much internalised his mother's punitive style and voice. Consequently, Daniel had difficulty applying self-care strategies, struggling to allow himself to rest, and resistant to allowing time to process loss. His response to the end of his relationship with Rebecca exemplified this.

"I can't stay there. As much as I want to, I can't," he shook his head. "I just want to curl up in a duvet on my mum's bedroom floor and lay next to her bed. But I know she wouldn't have that."

I just want to curl up in a duvet on my mum's bedroom floor and lay next to her bed. But I know she wouldn't have that.

There it was, the core of Daniel's distress. It was the most profound statement in all of our work together. I wanted to capture this moment, drill down on this thought.

"Tell me more about that, Daniel . . ."

"Just that. It's the only place I want to be. But I know she wouldn't let me. I don't even need her to say anything. I just want to know that she's there. I don't want be in a room on my own tonight, I don't want to be at my house on my own. I just want to be near her, be with her."

"I wonder if some of this distress about Rebecca also comes back to those feelings about your Mum. A yearning to be close to her, but knowing that you might be rejected?" I offered.

"Might be rejected?! I definitely *would* be." Pain echoed in his voice. The vulnerable part of Daniel had been exposed.

"That's a powerful image, Daniel. Wanting to be curled up on the floor next to your mum, but knowing she wouldn't allow it . . ."

Daniel interrupted me, jutting in quickly with a sharp change of tone. "I don't want to go into that stuff about my mum, thanks Freud. What are you going to say next, that it's really my mum that I want to sleep with? That wacky Oedipal stuff?" He reclined on the couch, mimicking the chaise longue position ubiquitous with Freud and psychoanalysis.

This seemed an invitation to delve deeper, disguised as a plea to keep the conversation shallow. A way to avoid the deeper hurt that would come from further discussion about his mother.

Despite my strong thoughts about the usefulness of exploring the relationship with his mother, I respected Daniel's overt wish of wanting to focus on the here-and-now, his current distress, and the relationship break-up with Rebecca. Pushing my agenda risked flooding Daniel with overwhelming feelings of shame and humiliation. Neither Daniel's ego nor our therapeutic relationship was well-developed enough to withstand that.

I was surprised to see Daniel in the waiting room the following week. He had not taken his usual place in my consulting room. Moreover, we didn't have an appointment scheduled.

I ushered my patient into my consulting room, returning to the waiting room and leading Daniel into an unoccupied room.

"Daniel, I don't think we have an appointment scheduled . . .?"

"No, but I need to see you. I need to see you now. I'm ready to come to sessions. I'm ready to book them all in. Sign me up! I'll attend weekly, daily . . . whatever you think I need! Weekends – do you do Saturdays? Please."

Daniel sat on the floor, legs crossed, head in hands. He grabbed a blanket from the couch and wrapped it around himself.

"I'm about to go into an appointment. Wait here and I'll come and collect you in an hour."

"Can't you just see me now? That other woman looked fine. Definitely a 'champagne problems' kind of person. She can wait."

"Wait here and I'll be back in an hour," I repeated. "Go and help yourself to a coffee from the kitchen. I'll be back."

I had enforced a boundary with Daniel. But was it too little, too late?

I turned and glanced at Daniel as I closed the door. Curled up on the floor, blanket draped haphazardly around him. He seemed smaller. An unguarded, shrunken version of the tall and strapping man I knew. I thought of Daniel wanting to be curled up next to his mother's bed, desperately seeking her approval and acceptance.

I felt a pressure to help Daniel. It seems I had been one of several women in his life to whom he turned to alleviate his excruciating feelings of distress. I wondered whether my experience was similar to Rebecca's, and that of other women in his life. A pressure to solve Daniel, to rescue him. Daniel had not experienced security and containment from his mother. Now, his attempts to establish and maintain relationships were immature and narcissistic, shielding from others his deep inner pain and his yearning for something more.

I returned to the room an hour later, as promised. The blanket was folded neatly on the couch. An empty coffee mug sat on the table.

I telephoned Daniel. No answer. I was considering calling the acute mental health care team to alert them to a man in the community who may be at risk, when I received a text message from Daniel: *I'm fine. I'm not going to do anything stupid. Just need some space. Catch you again some time.*

I saw Daniel many years later. He was alighting from a train, stumbling across the platform. His stained t-shirt and low-slung jeans incongruent with the chill of the cool Melbourne morning. He looked gaunt; the light behind his kind eyes somehow dimmed.

I watched Daniel as he staggered away, sauntering through the turnstile without swiping a ticket. My heart dropped. I had been harbouring hope, willing that his disengagement from our sessions was, against all odds, an indication of improved engagement and better fortune in his own life.

In retrospect, I had acted similarly to other women in Daniel's life. Allowing lax boundaries, letting him set the terms of our engagement and therapeutic relationship. I had been reactive, rather than providing the structure he needed. I had been charmed by Daniel's seemingly easy-going nature, his playful flirtation. His initial confidence was masking deep vulnerability and underlying narcissism.

I thought too about how the therapeutic relationship with Daniel had mirrored other relationships with men in my life. Flirtatious, charming, flattering. But in the final analysis, just like Daniel, many of the men were not who I thought or wanted them to be.

Daniel yearned for closeness and commitment, but this was unnatural and unfamiliar to him. He bristled, pushed it away, then rued missed opportunity. This process reinforced Daniel's self-belief of feeling unlovable, unworthy of attachment in the form of a stable partner. Thus, his ongoing internal conflict. As Oscar Wilde once stated: "There are only two tragedies in life: one is not getting what one wants, and the other is getting it."

FURTHER READING

Beattie, M. (2022). *Codependent no more: How to stop controlling others and start caring for yourself.* Spiegel & Grau.

Behary, W. T. (2021). *Disarming the narcissist: Surviving and thriving with the self-absorbed* (3rd ed.). New Harbinger Publications.

Jung, C. G. (2013). *The psychology of the transference.* Taylor and Francis.

Kottler, J. A. (2010). *On being a therapist* (4th ed.). Jossey-Bass.

Lavin, M., & Holowchak, M. A. (2018). *Repetition, the compulsion to repeat, and the death drive: An examination of Freud's doctrines.* Lexington Books.

McWilliams, N. (1999). *Psychoanalytical case formulation.* Guilford Press.

Perel, E. (2006). *Mating in captivity: Unlocking erotic intelligence* (1st ed.). Harper.

Sperry, L. (2016). *Handbook of diagnosis and treatment of DSM-5 personality disorders: Assessment, case conceptualization, and treatment* (3rd ed.). Routledge.

Winnicott, D. W. (with Winnicott, C., Shepherd, R., & Davis, M.). (2014). *Home is where we start from: Essays by a psychoanalyst.* W.W. Norton & Company.

Wolynn, M. (2017). *It didn't start with you: How inherited family trauma shapes who we are and how to end the cycle.* Penguin Books.

Yalom, I. D. (2017). *The gift of therapy: An open letter to a new generation of therapists and their patients* (reissued). Harper Perennial.

3

PETER PERFECT

If you really want to communicate something, even if it's just an emotion or an attitude, let alone an idea, the least effective and least enjoyable way is directly. It only goes in about an inch. But if you can get people to the point where they have to think a moment what it is you're getting at, and then discover it, the thrill of discovery goes right through the heart.

Stanley Kubrick

"I haven't heard anything from Peter in ten days. *Ten days!* No replies to my messages. I've tried to call him, no answer. I went to his house. The woman who answered the door said she has never heard of anyone called Peter. I told her there must be some mistake, maybe they know him by another name?"

Hannah reported the facts of her contact (or lack thereof) with Peter as if she was reading a pre-prepared statement. Monotonal voice. No emotion, no change in facial expression. She was motionless, her impeccable make-up undisturbed, not even a strand of hair out of place. She reminded me a little of a mannequin, wide-eyed and alert, but lacking substance.

"What do you make of all this?" I prompted gently.

"I guess he's just been too busy with work to return any of my messages. I know it's a really busy time for him. His job is really stressful at the moment, with the election coming up. I'm sure he will call when things settle down. Can you imagine how busy it must be for him at the moment?"

Peter seemed to be doing enough imagining for us all. It seemed clear as day – he was not who he said he was.

Hannah had achieved much in her professional life as a commercial lawyer. In this role, she had represented the taxation department in several major cases regarding tax fraud. Hannah had been the recipient of several awards for early career achievements in her field of taxation law. She was astute and careful in her work, her natural aptitude for numbers and rules lending itself well to the investigation and prosecution of fraudulent tax dealings.

DOI: 10.4324/9781003621645-4

Considerable professional achievements seemed to have come at the expense of Hannah's personal life. She had not married or had children, despite assuming from a young age that these would be central in her future.

Hannah's early life and family experiences informed much of her strong work ethic. The child of immigrants who had moved to Australia with little more than the clothes on their backs, Hannah's blue-collared parents had projected onto her their own unfulfilled academic and professional aspirations. She was aware that their investment in her education represented a huge sacrifice and the outcome of many years of hard toil. But, while praising her academic and professional achievements, Hannah's parents did little to hide their desire for grandchildren. Their expectation was that she fulfil the model of marriage and family. Hannah had long been expected to 'have it all' and 'do it all', a template that she had internalised and seemed to be bringing into her dating life.

In previous sessions, Hannah gushed about Peter. The compliments and platitudes poured out at such a rate that I wished I could turn off the metaphorical Tap of Peter. Finally, after years of being on the dating scene, Hannah had found her perfect match.

Peter ticked all Hannah's boxes. A professional man with a well-paid job. Good-looking and well-dressed. Not too short, not too tall. Courteous and polite. Intelligent and well-spoken.

Their initial dates had impressed Hannah. Expensive hotels, restaurants at which it was notoriously difficult to get a reservation, easy flowing conversation, and common interests. Their relationship moved quickly. At his encouragement, both Peter and Hannah deleted the dating app on which they had met; doing this in unison seemed a symbolic moment and a step towards the committed relationship Hannah had long yearned for. Moreover, he was up-front with his intentions – marriage and children. This was especially appealing for Hannah, aware of her age and mindful of the ticking of her biological clock.

Things cooled after the first few heady months of dating. The expensive hotels and fancy restaurants had given way to quieter nights in, usually at Hannah's apartment. An issue with Peter's phone meant Hannah always ordered and paid for the home-delivered meals. Soon after, daily communication dwindled to a few sporadic messages a week. He was busy, Hannah contended.

Hannah sought my reassurance that this end to the honeymoon period was normal.

"How do you feel about it, how does it feel to you?" I asked, careful to prompt reflection rather than provide a disingenuous response.

"He set a pretty high bar in those early days. I suppose that phase couldn't last forever."

"And how does that feel for *you*?" I prompted again, noticing Hannah had not mentioned her feelings, deflecting my direct question.

"I'm a bit flat about it. I mean, all that fancy stuff was really nice. I've never been treated like that before."

"Have you heard of the term 'love bombing'? Grand romantic gestures and intense displays of affection at the start of a relationship . . ."

"Well, they *were* grand. But now I just appreciate the small moments of time we do get to spend together."

"There's another term for that – 'breadcrumbing'. When you get just enough of something or someone – like when Peter stays for a few hours overnight – to keep you interested in him. Small things that leave a 'trail of breadcrumbs', leaving you wanting more, keeping you interested."

"Huh, maybe, but he's not like that . . ." Hannah answered abruptly.

I had come to understand Irvin Yalom's dislike for working with patients who are in love. He hated to be love's executioner; bringing those high on the endorphins of new love crashing back to earth with the reality-testing and introspection inherent to therapy.

Who was I to burst Hannah's love bubble? Her state of denial seemed so strong that I was not sure it could be queried, let alone penetrated or resolved. I was experiencing an internal conflict of my own: be a bystander to Hannah's naïvety, or risk being a messenger who may very well get shot.

I wondered what was underpinning my reaction to Hannah. It was not like me to shy away from hard truths with patients; I generally subscribed to the belief that a hard truth was better than a kind lie. I reflected on my own history of relationships and dating. Like most people, I've had my share of good and bad dating experiences. The horrible feeling of waiting for a reply to a message that never comes, finding a love letter to another women written by the person with whom I thought I was in a monogamous relationship, having a man tell me that he wasn't sure he could cope dating a woman whose salary exceeded his own. In those moments, would I have appreciated a hard truth or to continue with my naïvety? The thing that is the best for us in the long term often does not feel the best in the moment.

As senior staff to a federal politician, Peter had a fast and busy lifestyle. Constant travel, a demanding workload, receiving urgent phone calls and emails at all hours. Peter's time with Hannah was fleeting; he would often arrive late in the evening and leave before she woke. He often reminded her of the effort it took for him to make time and space to spend just a few hours with her. This seemed to have had its intended impact: Hannah felt special. An important person with a demanding schedule was prioritising her.

"Things will calm down after the election," Hannah purported to me, quickly adding that she secretly hoped Peter's boss would not hold his seat, as he could then get a 'normal job' that would better suit their relationship.

It all sounded too good to be true. And increasingly so, I thought it *was* too good to be true.

"What do your friends think of Peter?" I queried, attempting to encourage Hannah to consider a different perspective.

"Oh, they've not met him. They don't know anything about him. I mean, they know I've been seeing someone, but they don't know any of the details."

"He seems to have been a big part of your life over the past few months, I thought you would have been excited to share this with your friends?"

"It's his job. It's all pretty top-secret. He doesn't want anything getting out about his personal life, especially with the scandal around his boss earlier last year. Apparently, the media are always looking for dirt on politicians, and that extends to their staff, too. They are muckrakers, those journalists! Peter doesn't have any social media, not even a LinkedIn profile. And he's not listed on any government website, no profile there either. He said I could post about us on Instagram, as long as his face isn't visible. He thinks it's best to keep everything between us quiet for now, at least until after the election."

"That seems quite a feat in this day and age, to have no internet presence or electronic footprint," I mused. "And how do you feel about that, about keeping what's happening between the two of you low-key?"

"It's just for now. Just low-key for *now*. It won't always be like this. I would love to show him off to all my friends and family! But I know that will come. I just need to be patient. I've waited this long to find the right guy, I can wait a few more months for everything else to fall into place."

"He seems to be everything you've always wanted in a partner – intelligent, professional, good-looking . . . is there anything that has not 'ticked your boxes'?" I asked, borrowing Hannah's oft-used term.

"No, absolutely nothing. I can't quite believe it. It's like a shopping list where absolutely everything is in stock."

"How is that for you, feeling that you've finally found the perfect partner?"

"Thrilling. Just so exciting. I've never felt like this before. Finally, I feel like I've got the rest of my life to look forward to."

I was treading lightly. For a while I had wondered about Peter. He seemed to personify perfection. A mysterious and demanding job, keeping odd visiting hours, a reluctance to meet Hannah's friends, no electronic footprint, and an increasing avoidance of being seen in public with Hannah.

But, as any therapist knows, odd stories sometimes do add up. Reality can be stranger than fiction. Maybe Peter's circumstances *were* true. Perhaps his job did demand an extreme level of secrecy and conscientiousness regarding his public profile.

"I can understand how this relationship is really important to you, it has given you so much hope and excitement. It's still early days, you've got lots of time to get to know each other. You finding out a bit more about him, meeting each other's friends and family. Am I right in recalling that you've not been to his house yet?"

Hannah reminded me that she had seen his house once when she insisted on giving him a lift home. A beautiful double-fronted terrace in an affluent suburb. They had spoken about re-painting the exterior and getting a landscape gardener to re-design the 'disaster zone' that was the front yard. Peter was, of course, too busy to pay any attention to gardening. He promised to get onto it after the election. Hannah had searched the house online, wanting to see the floorplan to inform her thinking about interior design. She was surprised to find no online listing for the property, despite Peter's assertion that he had purchased it just a few years earlier. Another way to protect his privacy, Peter assured her, telling her it was usual amongst his colleagues to request the removal of online property listings after settlement.

"It seems like a lot is riding on this election, it seems this event is really shaping his life, and by extension, yours," I queried.

"I know. But I suppose politics is his life! He had politics long before he had me. I better get used to it!"

At the end of our session, I reminded Hannah that I would be on leave the following week.

"Oh, that's right!" she responded enthusiastically, "You're away for that conference. Are you all packed and ready to go?"

"No, not yet!" I replied, mindlessly adding, "I think I'm in denial about everything I need to do before I go!"

Hannah seemed oblivious to my unintentional mention of the word 'denial'. She wished me a safe trip, hoping I would catch some sun and have a chance to relax a little. She smiled broadly as she left the room, practically skipping through the door.

Upon my return from leave, Hannah told me that she had not heard from Peter for ten days. Ten days and nine hours, to be exact. And it was ten days, nine hours, and fifty minutes by the end of our session.

"I did something that I probably should not have done," Hannah started, staring at the floor rather than maintaining her usual eye contact.

"Go on," I encouraged gently.

"I know I wasn't meant to show anyone any photos of Peter. But I was just so excited that I couldn't help myself. I only showed one friend. Well, I sent her a screenshot of a photo of us, and she then showed it to a few of our other friends. I mean, I asked her not to! If she hadn't done that, maybe things would be different . . ."

"You told Peter this happened?"

"Yes, I had to. I felt really guilty for betraying his trust."

Oh, the irony, I thought to myself. Hannah feeling guilt for betraying the trust of this man who seemed to have been anything but truthful to her. Part of me wanted to tell her to run for the hills and forget she had ever met Peter, but I instead implored myself to sit with Hannah through this messy juncture.

"Let's go back a step, what happened when your friend saw the photo?"

"She thought he was handsome, a real catch. But then another friend said that she recognised him. She said he's still on the dating apps, but with a different name and new photos. She said his name there was Sam, and he listed his work as a pilot. His profile said he might take a few days to respond to messages, as he's often travelling."

"Oh, wow. That's a lot of information to take in. What do you make of it all?"

"I mean, maybe his name *is* Sam and maybe he *is* a pilot? Or maybe that's an alias he uses because he needs to keep his real job under wraps."

"But he's still on the dating apps, when you two deleted them together . . .?"

"It's probably just a glitch with the app. I mean, I *saw* him delete the app."

"But under a different name . . . how do we make sense of that?" I mused.

Silence.

"I don't know, but I know there must be an explanation for it all. He wouldn't do this to me. He wouldn't do this to *us*."

It was all too difficult, the idea of her fantasy not coming to fruition. Feeling her idea of happiness within her grasp, then losing it, was devastating. So devastating, in fact, that Hannah refused to accept it.

All the evidence consistently pointed in one clear direction: Peter was not the man he had presented himself to be. It seemed increasingly clear that he had deceived Hannah. Yet her reluctance to accept the truth was thus far unwavering.

We deny many things in life. The death of a loved one. The problematic nature of our drinking or substance use. The health impacts of our cigarette habit.

This is our attempt to avoid uncomfortable realities. Grief, the finality of death, distressing or painful solutions, or the reality of unpleasant events. A defence mechanism, our psyche's attempt to protect us from the hurt and distress that we are not equipped to manage. Denial is distinct from confabulation or not telling the truth; in those situations, people are aware of the truth but are consciously saying otherwise. Denial is a repression of the truth, not a mis-telling of it.

Some factors predispose us to engaging in states of denial. The capacity to cope with distress, our support systems, and the severity of the loss at stake. The stakes were high for Hannah. She had fulfilled her parents' wishes with her professional achievements, and in Peter had seen the possibilities to fulfil her ideal – or perhaps more accurately, her parents' ideal – of marriage and children.

"I met this guy, Mitchell. He's nice. Our dates have been good. But he's not Peter. I guess I'm just never going to find someone as perfect as Peter."

"Tell me more about Mitchell," I prompted.

"He's fine, I suppose. He's very polite. Reliable. Messages me when he says he is going to. He sent me flowers, that was nice. But the flowers Peter sent were much nicer, a bigger bunch, better flowers. He knew my taste."

"It seems all roads lead back to Peter . . ."

"Yeah, he was perfect," Hannah sighed.

"Or, the idea of Peter was perfect," I added.

Denial is hard to recognise, and even harder to shift. It seemed we still had much more work to do.

FURTHER READING

Behary, W. T. (2021). *Disarming the narcissist: Surviving and thriving with the self-absorbed* (3rd ed.). New Harbinger Publications.

Kahr, B. (2013). *Life lessons from Freud*. Macmillan.

Perel, E. (2006). *Mating in captivity: Unlocking erotic intelligence* (1st ed.). Harper.

Schwartz, R. C. (2021). *No bad parts: Healing trauma and restoring wholeness*. Vermilion.

Winnicott, D. W. (with Winnicott, C., Shepherd, R., & Davis, M.). (2014). *Home is where we start from: Essays by a psychoanalyst*. W.W. Norton & Company.

Yalom, I. D. (2013). *Love's executioner and other tales of psychotherapy* (new ed.). Penguin Books.

4

IS MY THERAPIST ANNOYED AT ME?

Countertransference insinuates itself into every course of psychotherapy.

Irvin D. Yalom

Isabelle positively beamed about her appointment with the psychiatrist. The psychiatrist, she exulted, understood her like no other mental health clinician. He immediately appreciated Isabelle's complex family dynamics. He provided strategies to manage difficult interactions with her parents and siblings. He drew inferences between Isabelle's early family experiences and her current feelings about pregnancy and impending motherhood. And, in a marked shift from her previous reluctance to consider medication, Isabelle had commenced an anti-depressant soon after the appointment.

My immediate reaction was relief. I was pleased the rapport was good and that Isabelle seemed committed to continuing to see the psychiatrist during what was likely to be a difficult transition to parenthood.

But, as Isabelle continued to wax lyrical, I noticed a shift in my initial sensation. Relief was giving way to other feelings. I felt a little dismissed, superseded by Isabelle's recall of the fantastical psychiatry consult. Quite quickly, her idealisation of him began to feel like a denigration of me and our therapy. Our years of work together seemed to have been pushed aside. The hard slog of our therapeutic work – in which we had explored her family dynamics, beliefs and schemas about families and parenthood, interpersonal relationships, reluctance to start her own family – overlooked. I felt neglected, irritated, a trifle annoyed.

I assumed my referral letter to the psychiatrist had informed his session with Isabelle. The letter detailed Isabelle's family history, diagnostic information, formulation, and Isabelle's engagement in our therapeutic work. I toyed with the idea of mentioning this to Isabelle; weighing this up I reminded myself of the golden rule of self-disclosure: only do so when the disclosure would benefit the patient. I quickly realised the statement would serve only to stroke my own ego, and thus resisted the disclosure.

On one hand, I was pleased the psychiatrist seemed to agree with my diagnosis and formulation. It is always satisfying for work to be endorsed by a colleague. On the other, I felt in some way that my work with Isabelle had been deftly lifted. Years of difficult

DOI: 10.4324/9781003621645-5

work presented back to Isabelle in a neat little package. It seemed akin to reading a three-page summary of a Shakespeare text; of course, it is more palatable, but no doubt simplified and missing a certain *je ne sais quoi*.

The news of Isabelle's pregnancy came as a surprise, both to Isabelle and to me. Over the years of our therapeutic relationship, Isabelle had vacillated between steadfast opposition and ambivalence at her partner's suggestion of having children. She never demonstrated enthusiasm for the idea, refusing to let herself indulge in any fanciful thoughts about parenting or children. Often, the pendulum swing between opposition and ambivalence seemed predicated on the tempestuous dynamics within her own family of origin – the idea of motherhood shut down when things were difficult with her own mother, then a softening occurring when relations were more harmonious. This indecision and reactivity formed the basis of our work together, providing much therapeutic fodder.

Like all of us, Isabelle's concept of parenthood and family was firmly shaped by her own childhood and early experiences. From a young age Isabelle experienced parentification, whereby she held responsibilities within the family beyond those typically assigned to a child. For Isabelle, this included many practical tasks such as housekeeping and cooking, in addition to the responsibility for the emotional wellbeing of her parents and siblings. Isabelle's rationale for her hesitation around having children seemed logical: as a function of her own parentification during childhood, she had already experienced many of the burdens that come with parenthood. Isabelle was not enthused at the prospect of entering a world in which she would again shoulder others' dependence. Rather, she had created a new identity for herself, one with a heavy focus on academic and professional achievement.

Isabelle had experienced several episodes of depression since adolescence. For many people, these would be debilitating, but Isabelle's perseverance in continuing study and work through the lowest of moods seemed a reflection of her family's attitude to any hardship: never explain, never complain. She also reported symptoms of anxiety, mostly around familial relationships and ongoing caregiver burden. Stress associated with her demanding job had precipitated several periods of burnout; similar to many people's experiences of burnout, Isabelle was prone to throwing herself further into the minutiae of work and family affairs, rather than embracing much-needed rest and recuperation.

Isabelle often experienced severe physical symptoms of anxiety and panic, including nausea, increased heartrate, and breathing difficulties. Her steadfast rejection of her family doctor's suggestion of trialling SSRI medication to manage these symptoms informed my approach of minimising discussion around medication; although I, too, thought Isabelle would likely benefit from medication, I was careful not to push the issue, wary this may cause a rupture in our therapeutic relationship and potentially leave her without any professional support. Her stoicism around this issue seemed a further reflection of her upbringing and family background; mental illness was not recognised, help was neither asked for nor received, and expression of any vulnerability either ignored or chastised.

Prior to her pregnancy, I had encouraged Isabelle to consult a psychiatrist regarding medication. I thought appealing to her sense of respect for professionals and detail-oriented nature may be helpful. However, her recent pregnancy and decline in overall functioning incited me to again raise the topic.

Even during the early stage of her pregnancy, several issues were of concern. Previous major depressive episodes predisposed Isabelle to experience perinatal depression. She openly mused about the "monumental fuck up" of becoming pregnant, shocked at the ease of conception while surrounded by same-aged friends complaining of fertility problems. Rolling her eyes as she described friends "peeing on ovulation strips every five minutes" and forgoing holidays and house deposits in favour of costly IVF procedures, Isabelle seemed trapped by an odd reality in which her lack of fertility problems was mismatched with her desire for pregnancy.

She described a sense of disgust at the idea of a foetus growing inside her. This was at odds with the actions of other expectant mothers, who commonly know their exact stage of pregnancy to the day and whimsically describe foetal development in comparison to the shape and size of a fruit or vegetable. All of this was missing with Isabelle. Even the absence of morning sickness and other early physiological changes associated with pregnancy was taken as an indication of her failure as an expectant mother. The lack of illness also assisted in perpetuating her denial of pregnancy in the early months, citing the old wives' tale of nausea being an indication of the viability of a pregnancy.

Isabelle mentioned several times her anticipation of being admitted to a psychiatric unit following the baby's birth, hoping her partner would be competent in dealing with "the kid." (In reality, mothers and babies are invariably admitted together to mother-baby psychiatric units.) Her assumption that she would be separated from the infant – an idea that seemed to bring some pre-emptive relief – suggested an emerging dichotomous relationship with her baby. Isabelle was imagining life after the baby's arrival as a time of individualism and continued autonomy. This seemed a re-emergence of her ambivalence about becoming pregnant. Isabelle now seemed to be looking for an exit strategy. While biologically capable of being a mother, her distance from any sense of maternal identity suggested she did not feel equipped for the demands of motherhood. Even at this stage, there seemed a distinct lack of connection to the baby. I feared this would not change even as the pregnancy progressed, and that Isabelle would not transition into a period of 'primary maternal preoccupation'. Coined by renowned British paediatrician and psychoanalyst Donald Winnicott, 'primary maternal preoccupation' refers to the biological and psychological attunement between mother and infant. This process occurs in late pregnancy and extends into the first few weeks of the infant's life. During this time the mother becomes hyper-focused on pregnancy and her baby, enabling her to become oriented to meeting the needs of the child.

To my surprise, Isabelle accepted the referral to a psychiatrist. Pre-empting her concerns around the potential loss of our therapeutic relationship, I assured her that our sessions would be ongoing. The psychiatrist would advise on medication, and be able to manage any imminent concerns that may arise during pregnancy or following the baby's birth. Unspoken was my relief that the responsibility for Isabelle's psychological wellbeing – and the welfare of her baby – was now shared.

Boy, was I relieved. I hoped that her experience with the psychiatrist I recommended would be a positive one, knowing that good psychiatric care during pregnancy would likely be advantageous. Prevention is better than cure in mental health; this is especially true in perinatal mental health.

My mind kept returning to those feelings of discontent that had begun bubbling away during the session with Isabelle. I felt my thunder had been stolen. I wanted someone – Isabelle, the psychiatrist, someone else? – to know that it was my hard work that had helped Isabelle. I had assisted Isabelle to understand her family dynamics. Strategies for managing interactions with family members had been discussed ad nauseum. I was with her during the dozens of hours of therapy in which her thoughts and feelings about pregnancy had been explored. These thoughts played through my mind as I imagined a convivial psychiatry consult, Isabelle relaxed and engaged, receptive to the psychiatrist's presentation of my information as his own.

Upon reflection, I thought a few therapeutic processes were occurring.

First, Isabelle had moved some way towards accepting that she needed help. After all, nothing indicates urgency more than the growing belly of pregnancy. It is a reminder that time is of the essence – to organise the baby's room, pack the hospital bag, stock up on onesies and nappies. For some people, including Isabelle, the arrival of a new baby may further complicate relationships within families. In this way, pregnancy also provides an impetus to make plans around management of family dynamics.

Second, the psychiatrist presented the information in a different way. Perhaps the short, sharp formulation had captured Isabelle's attention in a manner that our long, drawn-out work over several years could not. Long-term therapy versus a review session, analogous to a full football game and the highlights reel, respectively.

Third, Isabelle was idealising the psychiatrist and their session. He was being perceived as both a panacea and a saviour. A magical fairy-tale ending. But with Isabelle in the early stages of pregnancy, this story had many chapters yet to be written. Her feeling of confidence was simplistic and somewhat regressed, returning to a child-like dichotomy of things being 'good' or 'bad'.

Last, I bristled at the notion of being superseded by a male psychiatrist. Was this a case of 'father knows best', a reflection of our society in which men are listened to while women are side-lined, or – at best – expected only to assist men? From a feminist perspective, I pondered how this scenario and my reaction to it may have differed had the psychiatrist been female.

More challenging was the reflection on what was occurring for me during the session with Isabelle.

I recapped the gamut of reactions – relief (Isabelle had finally connected with a psychiatrist), surprise (her positive reaction to the consult with the psychiatrist), annoyance (not getting credit for my work), eventually circling back to relief (this is the best outcome for Isabelle and her unborn baby).

During my yoga session that evening I failed miserably at following the instructor's direction of 'letting go' of thoughts weighing me down. This represented an internalised conflict; thoughts of obeying the authority of the yoga instructor were in battle with my feelings of being my own person who is able to make autonomous decisions and can make choices around the things to which I pay attention.

Time and time again I returned to one feeling: annoyance. Its intensity failed to fade. I continued to feel slighted. Annoyed at their good rapport, annoyed that I had not been given credit for her diagnosis and formulation, annoyed that I was not being recognised.

I was experiencing a form of countertransference. Defined here as the therapist's response to a patient's enduring relational patterns, countertransference is a normal but extraordinary process during which the therapist's own experiences and attitudes inform their attitude and treatment towards a patient. This is conceptually similar to transference, in which the patient projects their thoughts about another person or event onto their therapist. Both transference and countertransference are reflections of enduring relationship patterns, usually developed during early childhood experiences.

The interactions with Isabelle stirred something at some level of my psyche. The distress and discomfort that had come to the fore following her contact with the psychiatrist stayed with me long after the conclusion of our session. I could not put down these thoughts. Unable to leave the interaction in the consulting room, I looked within myself for a potential answer.

Something within the experience with Isabelle was reminiscent of other times in which I felt I had been overlooked, not given credit. I trawled my mind for other times I felt like this, from earlier childhood experiences to more recent times.

One particular childhood memory came to mind. The early years of primary school. A teacher was distraught after losing a diamond from her engagement ring. Our whole year level was commandeered to search for the missing diamond. A warm, late-spring day. Luminous green grass a result of the mix of heavy rain and intermittent sunshine typical for the season. Ninety students lined up across the sports oval. We were instructed to commando crawl across the grass. Eyes down, bums up. The Willy Wonka-esque reward of an icy-pole for the child who found the diamond was enough to capture the imagination and energy of the group of 8-year-old children. The child who found the diamond would also be presented with an award at a whole-school assembly. This combination of reward represented the highest accolade at our school.

The wave of crawling children reached the halfway point of the oval. Class clowns yelled false alarms, raising the ire of staff pulled from other classes to supervise the unusual school activity. The young teacher looked increasingly distraught. A slight figure standing to the side of the oval, her Farrah Fawcett hair dazzled in the sun. The principal wrapped a reassuring arm around the bereft young woman. One older teacher was militant in her command of the students, her distress second only to her younger colleague whose diamond was the centre of attention. I recalled a few years earlier that she had left a class distraught after the school principal had entered and asked quietly for her to join him. Her husband had died by suicide. Years later I connected the dots as to why this search held such importance for her.

I hoped I wouldn't find the diamond. I didn't want an icy-pole. I didn't want any attention on me. I was filled with dread at the idea of standing in front of the whole school, overwhelmed at the idea of receiving public praise.

What are the chances, I thought, of the diamond being found? What are the chances of *me* finding this diamond? Slim to none on both accounts, I silently reassured myself. Compliant nonetheless, my eyes were glued to the ground. I visually sifted through each blade of grass, alert for any glimmer in the late afternoon sun.

And then I saw it. I blinked slowly, hoping it was an apparition. But there it was: a diamond, no bigger than my fingernail, the sun bouncing off its acute edges.

I panicked. Part of me wanted to ignore the diamond. To keep crawling, to pretend I had never seen in. I was torn, wanting the young teacher to be reunited with her precious jewel, feeling pressure from the older teacher to meet her unspoken demand for this endeavour to be a success, but dreading the credit and acknowledgement that I would receive as a result of it. I now recognise this to be an early experience of internal conflict; I was grappling with the notion that two things can be concurrently true yet also seem to be in diametrical opposition. I turned to the boy next to me, Mark. Whispering his name, I pointed to the diamond. He grabbed it quickly, leaping up to proclaim his victory.

A palpable sense of relief spread across the group. High-fives among kids, hugs between teachers. I was relieved, but for a different reason – thrilled to have avoided the spotlight. Pleased for the teacher to be reunited with her diamond, but relieved to have not received credit for the find.

Later that afternoon, the canteen opened especially for the occasion of Mark receiving his icy-pole. A cheer among the school kids erupted as the roller door opened. Mark ran around the school yard, announcing how refreshing it was to have an icy-pole on such a warm day.

The following week, he strode with confidence across the stage at the school assembly, receiving his certificate from the principal. The whole incident was soon fodder for school-gate conversations and school community chatter, eventually entering school-yard folklore.

I kept quiet, experiencing what I now recognise to be conflicting emotions between not receiving credit while also feeling a sort of discomfort and resentment at the fanfare surrounding Mark.

At that time, I was not conscious of any feelings of envy. Rather, I felt relief that Mark had taken the credit. I was off the hook. I perceived his actions as a favour, removing me from the spotlight. In retrospect, I was likely inferring too much from this. My young self was wanting care and protection from Mark, when in reality his celebratory response may have been demonstrating nothing more than ego-centrism and self-centredness typical of a young boy.

The same cycle I have experienced time and time again in life was playing out once more. I did not attend any of the graduation ceremonies for the three university degrees I hold. I had to be convinced that walking down an aisle and having a photographer present was a normal and expected part of being the bride at my own wedding. I downplay my honorarium, reminding people who address me as 'Doctor' that I am not a medical doctor, joking that I can only be of assistance with people's feelings. I even thought twice about writing this very book, such is my anticipatory horror at the thought of receiving credit or praise for it, or, God forbid, being required to do promotion or attend my own book launch.

Doing the work, not requesting credit, then feeling resentment at the lack of acknowledgement. A lifelong pattern, playing out in my work as a therapist and coming alive time and time again in my therapeutic relationships with patients.

I thought of Ernest Hemingway's famous quote, imploring that one must always be prepared to work without applause. Had I read this as a child and adopted it as my unconscious mantra? Sure, there's honour in humility, but for me this seemed to be reaching a stage of counterproductivity. I began to wonder whether my humility was acting as a proxy for other internal processes.

Could I have projected (or transferred) my feelings onto the situation with Isabelle? My 'What about me?' mindset had been triggered once again, despite the logical part of my psyche knowing that the psychiatrist's success was not my failure. But in that moment, I was that little girl, watching Mark collect his icy-pole, watching him receive credit and acknowledgement for my actions.

A couple of years after the great diamond find, I was paired with Mark on a fundraising task. We door-knocked the local neighbourhood to raise funds for a charity. (The charity was the 40 Hour Famine; in late 1980s Australia it was *au fait* to encourage children to not eat for forty hours. Two unaccompanied primary-school-aged children door-knocking would also be frowned upon today!) Mark did all the talking. I stood a few steps behind, clutching the collection tin, stepping forward only to collect coins and mutter a quiet but sincere 'thank you'. I was convinced that Mark's charming manner and animated description of the charity was no doubt the reason for us topping the collection tally. Looking back, I again denigrated myself to the role of his subordinate.

We were due to receive a certificate at the whole school assembly in recognition of our fundraising efforts. I urged him to go ahead without me, telling him I had barely contributed. Mark took my hand, led me onto the stage towards the principal, whispering "you deserve this," and assuring me I would be alright. Perhaps he knew me better than I thought.

As an adult viewing this through a feminist lens, I see the gender trope at play – the boy saving the girl, the male leading the female. Did he know me better than I thought? Or did I, like Isabelle and the psychiatrist, idealise him as someone who could see me and save me? I had inserted Mark into that role in my mind to meet some unspoken need, just as Isabelle had with the psychiatrist.

An email landed in my inbox a few weeks after Isabelle's initial consultation.

> *Dear Bianca,*
>
> *Our mutual patient, Isabelle, speaks very highly of you. Thank you for your ongoing and valuable work with her.*
>
> *Do you have capacity to accept a new referral? The patient is a new mother experiencing anxiety after a difficult start with her infant. I believe she would benefit from psychotherapy with you.*

Noticing countertransference can be difficult. It is sometimes hard to see the forest for the trees. Therapists are not always insightful about their reaction to issues raised by or inferred through patients. These blind spots inevitably impact therapy and therapeutic outcomes, in both positive and negative ways. But problematic issues arise when these blind spots are not recognised or discussed. This can blindside therapists and patients alike, leading to therapeutic ruptures and suboptimal therapeutic outcomes.

Some instances of countertransference are easy to spot. I once walked into the waiting room to greet a new patient, and was shocked to see it was my ex-boyfriend. Well, it wasn't him, but a person who shared a striking physical similarity to him. Another time, a patient who was a police officer told me that intervention orders were usually instigated by bored housewives. He insisted that such orders were not "real police work." I recoiled at the notion, recognising the impact that my own experiences with family violence and the court system would have on our therapeutic relationship. For some patients I make special concessions or allowances (running over session time, squeezing in an after-hours appointment, loaning a book from my personal collection). This is likely a reflection of a conscious or unconscious recognition of a shared trait or characteristic between the patient and me.

With Isabelle, I also recognised countertransference coming from my own maternal experiences. I had made a special effort to source a respected psychiatrist for her, referring to a colleague with whom I thought Isabelle may connect well and who I was assured would provide quality psychiatric care. I had discussed Isabelle and her presentation in our peer supervision group; as I was describing my concerns, I realised that I felt more invested in Isabelle's wellbeing (and that of her unborn child) than I did with the problems presented by other patients. I want good care for all my patients, but with Isabelle this extended to a deeper level of *needing* good care. Perhaps this was a message from my subconscious that I felt something was lacking in my own experiences of perinatal care. This speaks to the positive aspects that can arise from countertransference; caregiving was elicited in me, based on my recognition of my own needs.

So, is your therapist annoyed with you? The more interesting question centres around why your therapist may be annoyed with you, and why it is that you may feel they are annoyed. These notions represent forms of countertransference and transference, respectively.

Was I annoyed with Isabelle? Perhaps it is more accurate to say that I was experiencing annoyance from previous events and interactions, and then projecting that annoyance onto my therapeutic relationship with Isabelle. The discomfort from the recognition of my own relational patterns played out throughout the therapeutic work with Isabelle, simmering away until brought into focus by my more overt reaction to Isabelle's experience with the psychiatrist.

Therapists are, of course, people. We have personal histories that shape perspectives and experiences of the world. This countertransference invariably impacts therapeutic work. The astute therapist, however, will recognise this and act accordingly.

FURTHER READING

Adams, M. (2024). *The myth of the untroubled therapist* (2nd ed.). Routledge.

Delft, F. van. (2012). *Transference and countertransference: A therapeutic method for application in everyday psychosocial counseling*. Eleven International Publishing.

Gabbard, G. O. (2005). *Psychodynamic psychiatry in clinical practice* (4th ed). American Psychiatric Pub.

McWilliams, N. (1999). *Psychoanalytical case formulation*. Guilford Press.

McWilliams, N. (2011). *Psychoanalytic diagnosis*. Guilford Press.

Quatraro, R. M. & Grussu, P. (eds). (2020). *Handbook of perinatal clinical psychology: From theory to practice* (English edition). Routledge.

Schwartz, R. C. (2021). *No bad parts: Healing trauma and restoring wholeness*. Vermilion.

Seu, I. B. (ed.). (1998). *Feminism and psychotherapy: Reflections on contemporary theories and practices*. Sage.

Winnicott, D. W. (1998). *Babies and their mothers*. Addison-Wesley Publishing.

Winnicott, D. W. (with Winnicott, C., Shepherd, R., & Davis, M.). (2014). *Home is where we start from: Essays by a psychoanalyst*. W.W. Norton & Company.

Yalom, I. D. (2013). *Love's executioner and other tales of psychotherapy* (new ed.). Penguin Books.

Yalom, I. D. (2017). *The gift of therapy: An open letter to a new generation of therapists and their patients* (reissued). Harper Perennial.

5

DEATH BECOMES HER

Life can only be understood backwards, but it must be lived forwards.

Sören Kierkegaard

Death will come to us all. Existential psychotherapy theory and practice posits that much anxiety stems from this inevitability. Perhaps contrary to common belief, it is not the process of death or dying itself that induces fear. Rather, existential dread is fuelled by the notion of living an unfulfilled life. It is not dying that we fear, but instead dying with regret.

Lee, a 59-year-old woman, was admitted to the palliative care ward following a recurrence of pancreatic cancer. Referral information stated that Lee was highly distressed, particularly in the evenings and overnight. Her aggressive behaviour and verbal outbursts were increasingly disruptive to other patients.

I entered the palliative care ward with some trepidation. I had very little personal or professional experience with death and dying. The ward was like any other in the hospital, albeit a little quieter and featuring a softer colour scheme and décor.

It was a striking mid-autumn day, glistening leaves starting to turn to deeper colours, the chill in the air balanced by bright sunshine. I thought about the patients on the palliative care ward, that this would be the last autumn they would experience. They had enjoyed their last Christmas and many would not celebrate another birthday. Final goodbyes to their loved ones were imminent.

I heard Lee before I saw her. She was shouting at the TV, seemingly frustrated by the glitchy remote control.

"Love," she addressed me abruptly, "do us a favour and switch the channel from this garbage."

I complied with her order, scanning through the limited channels until we landed on something to her liking. She begrudgingly agreed to my suggestion of lowering the volume while we chatted. Next up, I was to help her with a crossword. Her eyesight, she explained, was letting her down, and she could no longer complete it without assistance.

DOI: 10.4324/9781003621645-6

And so, our therapeutic relationship began over a crossword. Between crossword clues we spoke of her experiences of psychological distress during her admission, her symptoms of panic, and difficulties with other patients and staff.

"*Of course* I'm anxious, I'm bloody well dying!" Her candour was both refreshing and confronting. The elephant in the room had been addressed. Lee would not be leaving this ward. This was the end of her life.

Lee averted her gaze, avoiding eye contact. The distant sound of the lunch trolley prompted her to speculate on today's meal, commenting that she hoped it wouldn't be as bad as yesterday's.

"I'm tired now, but you can come back tomorrow," Lee instructed.

I wrote up my notes, reporting her symptoms, including a plan for the nurses to respond to Lee when in a state of distress. I pondered the plan for our next session. We had discussed Lee's symptoms and ascertained the normality of these given her terminal illness. However, I knew there was so much yet to learn about Lee and her life. I felt there was a piece of the puzzle missing. This is often the case during initial sessions of therapy; more is revealed as therapeutic rapport is established, with the patient feeling increasingly comfortable to reveal their personal history and inner-most thoughts.

A nurse approached me. A look of apprehension on her kind face. In a whispered tone she expressed exasperation at Lee's behaviour. Lee, she reported, was extremely anxious when visitors left, insisting her partner or children be present at all hours. While visiting hours in palliative care were more extensive than in other wards, Lee's demands were disruptive to staff and other patients, with some families complaining about the interruption to time with their own loved ones. Further, Lee's family members reported emotional and physical exhaustion, feeling torn between staying by her bedside and returning home for much-needed respite. No amount of attention or company seemed sufficient to soothe Lee. In some moments, the nurse reported, Lee would act like a young girl. Her voice would rise to a high pitch, at times she would suck her thumb, tantrum like a toddler, push her food tray onto the floor if the meal was not to her liking. Lee was regressing to a child-like state.

I was starting to build a formulation in my mind about the factors informing Lee's distress, beyond her self-assessment of anxiety associated with terminal illness. The information from the nurse provided some additional pieces of the formulation puzzle. The regressed behaviour, separation anxiety, and abrupt nature were all similar to the temperament of a young child. In the absence of being able to verbally articulate her thoughts and feelings, Lee had resorted to child-like behaviour.

I hypothesised that Lee had experienced trauma in her life, most likely in her early years. The unresolved trauma was the impetus for ongoing psychological distress. This, I thought, had given way to her current expression of existential pain.

We switched from crosswords to Scrabble in our next session. The first player to reach 100 points was declared the winner, the expedited game owing to Lee's fatigue and increasingly short concentration span. "You're a clever one, aren't cha?!" she would say with a wink and glint in her eye when I placed a high-scoring word.

The game provided a gentle space to discuss Lee's childhood and family background. Lee was raised in abject poverty, one of a gaggle of children who endured abuse and parental neglect. She reported her father to be a chronic alcoholic, with most of the family's meagre income spent at the local pub. Lee reflected on walking miles to school, chronic hunger amidst a paucity of food, clothes handed down between children until in a state of absolute disrepair, committing petty theft from the local store to gain access to necessities. She indicated being the victim of both sexual and physical violence within the family home, feeling unprotected by any adult during her childhood.

Lee had been estranged from her family for most of her adult life. In her own words, she "hightailed it out of there as soon I could." Lee's children and partner had not met her parents or siblings. Intermittent contact with one sibling provided a conduit for information: both parents were alive, however her father had been diagnosed with dementia several years earlier.

Lee recalled the details of her life with little emotion. She reeled off the facts as if reading a charge sheet. No point dwelling on the past, she said. She had learned to separate herself from her family and early experiences, building a new life not contingent on her childhood. I reflected to Lee the courage and fortitude she demonstrated in creating a life away from the glare of her family and the shadow of its trauma. There is a sense of pride and joy from making your own way in the world, but this can also be coupled with a great sense of responsibility and feelings of being unsupported and untethered. As she nodded softly in agreement, I noticed a passing look of sadness, a change from her usual hardened expression. I wondered if my empathic response was novel for her. Had others sympathised or commiserated about the abuse and trauma she endured? Were others even aware of her experiences? Lee had a tough exterior and was nobody's fool, but in that moment a softness had crept in. A glimpse of the little girl who had found her own way through life, who had no safe place to land within her family, who felt betrayed by the very people meant to care for her.

People generally hold an intellectual acknowledgement of adverse events. Bad things do happen. We read about these events in newspapers and hear the names of victims on news reports. But most of us are safe in the assumption that those bad things happen to other people. This is a superficial but effective defence mechanism; we engage in this world thinking that we are safe, taking chances and living our lives under the premise that we will be treated fairly.

Individuals who have experienced trauma often adopt a different perspective. Trauma survivors maintain an acute awareness that bad things *do* happen, that bad things *have* happened, and that bad things *will* occur again. Many people who have experienced trauma develop a hypervigilance to risk, a false alarm that signals terror in response to innocuous stimuli. In fact, trauma survivors greatly overestimate their chance of experiencing adverse events. They experience a foreshortened sense of future, and often believe they are plagued with misfortune and bad luck. Amongst survivors of trauma there is an inherent awareness of the cruelty of the world, the reality of there being no safety net in this life.

The past was not as far below the surface as Lee may have wished. I theorised her current experiences – panic attacks, verbal outbursts, difficulties with staff and other patients – were a result of the life events on which she had consciously not dwelled. I shared this with Lee.

"Sometimes," I explained, re-arranging my Scrabble tiles on the wooden rack before pausing to make eye contact with Lee, "distress can be a bit like pushing a beachball under the water. The harder we push it down, the more pressure it causes, and the bigger the splash when the beachball finally slips out of our hands." I emphasised the point by pushing down an imaginary object, then throwing up my hands as if releasing handfuls of confetti.

I saw the hint of tears welling in Lee's eyes. This hardened woman, accustomed to brushing aside her own feelings in the pursuit of pragmatism, was again displaying emotion. In that moment I again saw Lee as a little girl. I thought of her experiences of hunger, of being teased at school for being barefoot, of her terror of being left alone at night. A child whose basic needs were never met, giving no opportunity for higher order needs or emotional wellbeing to be considered. The hurt had never been resolved. Lee had developed a thick skin to protect her from revisiting this pain. Her abrupt nature and domineering personality were warning signs to others, barriers to people getting too close, a blockade to people who could potentially cause more pain, a buffer against recalling the pain endured in childhood. *I'll scare you away before you scare me*, her actions seemed to scream.

A shift occurred. Something in the space between us changed. Just for a moment, I felt Lee let me in to her internal world. One of pain, hurt, abandonment, fear, rejection. I held her gaze as a solitary tear dropped down her cheek. I leaned forward and put my hand on hers. After a few minutes I gently pushed my chair back, setting the Scrabble board aside while being careful to maintain the position of the letter tiles. I quietly told a sleepy Lee that I would see her the following day.

The contemplative mood seemed to have passed overnight. Lee seemed spritely, energised. I wondered for a moment if I had imagined yesterday's overt vulnerability and change in affect, so far removed it seemed from her current state.

"Sit down, love. No Scrabble today, let's get down to business." She pulled herself up to a seated position in bed, wincing with pain as she settled back onto her pillow.

"Write this down," she instructed.

I promptly pulled up a chair and poised my notebook and pen.

Lee expressed two clear aims for our work together. First, to reunite with her family before her upcoming sixtieth birthday. Second, to receive an apology from her family for the lack of love received during her childhood.

My pen hovered over the page. I felt bamboozled at the gravity of these requests. Family estrangement offers challenging terrain for therapists. Lee's terminal illness added a layer of complexity. I was still processing this information, formulating some kind of response, when Lee dropped a bombshell: her family would be visiting the following afternoon. The visit had been coordinated with her sister's assistance. Lee informed me that I would be facilitating the meeting. I wondered if her sister's cooperation had been similarly harangued.

"I'll see you then, love," she offered quickly, before telling me to book the common room for the following afternoon. She settled back into her bed. The end of our conversation was signalled by Lee pulling up her bedsheets and closing her eyes.

"I'll be there, see you then," I farewelled Lee, surprising myself with the conviction in my voice.

Lee was in charge of our therapeutic relationship. From the outset of our work together she called the shots. The relationship between a therapist and patient – what happens between the two people in a therapy room (or, in this case, beside her hospital bed) – provides a wealth of information that informs the therapist's formulation and understanding of their patient. The forthright way in which she led our therapeutic relationship indicated Lee was a person accustomed to being in charge. Terminal illness no doubt robbed her of some of that sense of control and reduced her capacity to lead her own life. In such moments, it seemed, Lee regressed to her child-like state, seeking the help and care she had been deprived of during childhood. Her self-sufficiency was born out of necessity. A need to rely on herself, having experienced disappointment and rejection from those entrusted with her care.

The following day I found myself again walking into the ward with a sense of trepidation. Running through my head were the scenarios of what may unfold in the family meeting. I thought about Lee's parents – the violent alcoholic father and negligent mother – and made a conscious effort to suppress my assumptions and negative feelings.

I considered the best way to enter the common room. While Lee was my patient and I was clear about my role in advocating for her, I was acutely aware of the need to present neutrality in order to facilitate rapport with all family members and enable a constructive conversation.

I spied the family through the glass doors of the common room. I hovered a little longer than intended; perhaps this was an indication of my reluctance to enter the room and risk becoming central to the family fray. An elderly man, whom I assumed was Lee's father, was slumped in a wheelchair. Mouth agape and eyes fluttering shut, he seemed unaware of his surroundings. An older woman, her hand gripping the arm of the man's wheelchair. Broad-shouldered and grey-haired, pain etched into the lines on her face. Her eyes darted around the room, as if in the principal's office waiting to be reprimanded. Two younger women, presumably Lee's sisters, sat nearby.

Lee entered the room, wheeled in by a nurse. Her partner and children traipsed behind, looking downcast and awkward.

"Well, look what the cat dragged in!" Lee's attempt at breaking the ice fell flat. Her mother and sisters remained stony-faced. Lee's mother bristled as her daughter entered the room, the hostile reaction reminiscent of Lee's strained interactions with some staff and patients. Her father's state of oblivion continued.

I entered the room soon after Lee, introducing myself and inviting everyone to take a seat. I observed the position in which the family members sat. This can give an indication of the relationships within families, marking alliances and estrangements. In longer-term family therapy, re-positioning family members can facilitate interactions and communication between family members which may not otherwise occur.

Lee instructed the nurse to wheel her to the space at the head of the table. Her sisters and parents sat at opposite sides of the table. I scanned the group and formulated a genogram (family tree) in my mind. Two separate alliances between parents and sisters, indicated by their paired seating. Lee placing herself in charge of the group, with her family having left the head-of-table spot available. Lee's partner and teenage children sat back from the group, seemingly symbolic of their long-held ostracisation from the family. They declined my invitation to join the table with a collective emphatic shake of their heads.

Although relatively ad hoc, the family meeting provided an opportunity for a systemic intervention. The systemic approach acknowledges that problems are not based in the individual, but rather in the system in which the individual functions. In this case, Lee's distress could be viewed as a reaction to her place in the family and her experiences of the way in which the family system operated. One way of viewing family systems is that one plus one does not equal two; rather, it equates to three – the two people involved plus the space between them. Multiply this by several family members and the complexity of family relationships and dynamics quickly becomes evident.

A systemic therapist is mindful of many levels of interactions and communication between family members, some of which are overt and others more discreet. In this case, several concepts of systemic intervention were at play; already observable were alliances (a collection or union of family members who share a mutual interest) and coalitions (a dysfunctional alliance between two or more family members). I was acutely aware of my need to join the family (through making a connection and establishing therapeutic rapport) while not isolating any one person or sub-group of people.

I asked permission of the family to set ground rules for the gathering. Each agreed to respect others' time to speak, to take turns to speak, to not interrupt, and to avoid inflammatory and abusive language.

I invited Lee to start the conversation. Her physical pain was obvious, grimacing as she re-positioned herself in the wheelchair. She closed her eyes for a few moments and took a few deep breaths. Lee's eyes flickered open. She spoke quietly but clearly.

"I've called you here today, because . . ." she sighed before a long pause. I scanned the room: her father oblivious, mother angry, sisters anxious and upset, partner and children avoidant. I wondered if this was exemplary of their usual family dynamic.

"I want to set a few things straight. I'm on my way out and I need to set a few things right. My childhood was *shitty*. You," Lee began, slowly raising a finger to point at her mother, "treated us horribly. I want you to acknowledge what I went through, what we all went through."

Silence. Lee's mother rolled her eyes. Her father maintained his absent stare. The sisters stared at the ground, looking as if they wished to be swallowed up by it.

"I want an apology," Lee continued, apparently undeterred (or, perhaps motivated) by the lack of any reciprocity in the conversation thus far. Her voice was rising in volume, her confidence seemingly increasing.

Her mother was vicious in response. "Listen here," she spat, "we did the best we could with all you kids. Do you think it was easy for us? All you kids, no money. We. Did. The. Best. We. Could."

She continued, seething as she spoke through clenched teeth. She accused Lee of putting her father through hell, of dragging him here at this stage of his illness. He gave a vague glance at the recognition of his name. Couldn't she just let things lie? Why drag up the past now? Lee's mother said the times were different, life was different then, they were no different to other local families.

Lee fought back, her voice and tone eerily similar to her mother's. She demanded an apology, an acknowledgement of the truth. She told them she wanted to be told that she was loved. Her harsh tone seemed inconsistent with the heartfelt plea.

A fiery stare between mother and daughter. Two strong personalities, two people for whom anger and aggression had become a default defensive position.

I worried that this meeting was only making matters worse for Lee. It is one thing to be estranged from your family at the time of your death, it is another for it to end with demonstrable acrimony.

I suggested we take a break, as much for me to strategise a way forward as to give the family members a much-needed breather. An overwhelmed Lee asked her daughter to take her to the bathroom. A silence settled over the group. Lee's sister spoke for the first time, pleading with her mother in a hushed tone to apologise to Lee, to give Lee what she needed.

Tears welled in her mother's eyes. Another softening of another hardened woman.

"I'm just not ready yet," she whispered, staring at the tabletop.

I felt a pang in my chest. Families are not black and white, people are neither good nor bad, there were no villains or victors here. Everyone was hurting. Each person in this room had found a way to cope with a lifetime of distress, to cope with the dysfunction of their family. Avoidance, anger, humour, deflection, blame. Labelling a coping strategy as adaptive (helpful) or maladaptive (unhelpful) is a simplistic construct; those strategies developed in a time of need and served a purpose at that time. A coping strategy is neither good nor bad. Objectively, smoking is bad; subjectively, it may help an individual cope with a traumatic event, preventing them from engaging in more harmful behaviour. Sometimes, however, strategies continue to be applied beyond their usefulness; this may often be an indication of the enduring nature of the trauma or difficulty which the coping strategy was developed in response to.

I thought of Lee's mother, of the dreams she likely once held for her children. No one enters into parenthood hoping their final interaction with their child will be a terse conversation on a palliative care ward.

I gently reminded her of the nature of Lee's terminal illness. She closed her eyes and placed her face in her hands. Lee re-entered the room.

And then, an unexpected moment, one of clarity and beautiful insight.

"Of course, we've always loved you."

It was Lee's father, breaking his silence in the most poignant way. He suddenly looked vibrant, alive, sitting upright and looking directly at Lee. His energy and attention seemed to pass as quickly as its onset. He slumped back into his chair and gazed into the distance. The family were silent in their mutual shock, giving way to a cascade of tears. Lee's mother stood up and embraced her daughter. The sisters joined, each vying for physical closeness with Lee.

I pushed my chair away from the table and quietly relocated to the window. I paused for a few moments, watching this reunion unfold. Lee called her children over, their grandmother embracing them for the first time.

I attempted to give the family a modicum of privacy by directing my attention to the scene outside the window. The common room was on the third floor, providing a serene view of surrounding trees. The blanket of autumn colour had started to thin, leaves dropping to the ground, giving way to bare patches amongst the canopy. I thought about the passage of time, of the vibrant colours of those trees when I had first met Lee. I had felt overwhelmed by her plight, pressured to fix what seemed irreparable. But looking at those trees with the din of Lee and her family in the background, I realised something about my own distress related to Lee: I had felt the need to control the situation, the pressure to provide some kind of remedy, to put everything in its rightful place before her death.

I had learnt that nothing is really within our control, especially when the dynamics of individuals and families are at play. It was my job to provide a space for Lee to do what she always knew she needed to do, just as the autumn weather provided the conditions for what those trees knew they always needed to do. Lee and her family had dropped their guards, just as those trees were dropping their leaves. Trust in people, trust in seasons, trust in time.

I quietly left the room and found a space at the nurse's station to write my notes. A few minutes later I saw Lee and her mother careening around the corridors of the ward, her mother deftly controlling the wheelchair, pausing every few metres at Lee's request. The scene was reminiscent of a toddler in a stroller; any parent will tell you that the parent pushes the stroller but the toddler is very much in charge. Lee showed her mother around the ward that had been her home for several weeks. The interactions between mother and daughter reminded me of a child having their parent accompany them on a school excursion. The young child bursts with pride to have their parent present, provides introductions, feels a sense of ownership, and is pleased to connect their parent to this part of their life.

Lee celebrated her sixtieth birthday the following week. The party was a great success, with Lee able to take day leave from hospital to gather with family and friends at home.

Lee proudly showed me photos from the day. One in particular struck me. I returned to it as we reached the end of the printed stack of images. Lee, sitting wide-eyed in front of her birthday cake. In that photo I again saw that little girl. A little girl who had likely not experienced her own birthday parties in childhood. This was her opportunity to be the birthday girl, to revel in her family celebrating her, to experience the fun and frivolity of birthdays denied in her younger years. She had her cake and ate it too.

I returned to the ward the following week. The chill of winter had truly set in. The last of the patchy autumn leaves were gone, replaced with bare trees and grey skies. Despite the gloomy weather, I had a spring in my step, thinking about the remarkable outcome of the family session and feeling vicariously buoyed by the joy of Lee's birthday party. I was looking forward to seeing Lee. I had brought the newspaper, hoping we might have a chance to complete the crossword together.

Lee was sitting up in bed, staring blankly at the wall. Her gaze unmoved as I approached. Lee did not recognise me. She stared through me, her face reminding me of her father's during our family meeting. She smiled softly as her eyes fluttered shut.

I sat with her for a brief moment, leaving the newspaper on her bedside table. I knew that would be the last time we saw each other. My note in her file that day indicated she was no longer able to participate, and hence psychological treatment was terminated.

Lee was still alive, but already gone to me. I felt a sense of loss. I sat in the garden courtyard for a few minutes after leaving the ward. It was empty, owing to the cold weather and imminent rain. I thought about the grief I was experiencing for Lee, for our short but meaningful relationship. For a moment I chastised myself for feeling upset – Lee was my patient, not my friend. These tears belonged to her family and friends, not me. But I stopped and let myself feel exactly what came – the thought that I am a human grieving for another human. Grief is not a competition; my grief was no doubt different from that experienced by others in Lee's life, but nonetheless remained genuine and deeply felt.

The following day I logged onto the hospital system and searched Lee's record. Deceased. Two weeks after the reunification with her family, a week after her sixtieth birthday.

I am forever grateful for the experience of working with Lee and her family. I often think of her, especially as the leaves are changing colour and the majestic red and orange autumnal tones turn to bare trees and dark skies.

Our work together reinforced the notion that no patient is beyond being helped. All patients deserve care regardless of their stage of life or circumstances. The care provided for people at their end of life, a time at which they are often at their most vulnerable both psychologically and physically, epitomises humanity.

FURTHER READING

Gostečnik, C. (2017). *Relational family therapy: The systemic, interpersonal, and intrapsychic experience.* Routledge.

Hackney, H. L., & Cormier, S. (2009). *The professional counselor: A process guide to helping*. Merrill.

McWilliams, N. (1999). *Psychoanalytical case formulation*. Guilford Press.

Minuchin, S. (2003). *Families and family therapy* (29th ed.). Harvard University Press.

Rogers, C. R. (2004). *On becoming a person: A therapist's view of psychotherapy*. Constable.

Samuel, J. (2022). *Every family has a story: How we inherit love and loss*. Random House Canada.

Van der Kolk, B. A. (2015). *The body keeps the score: Mind, brain and body in the transformation of trauma*. Penguin Books.

Winnicott, D. W. (with Winnicott, C., Shepherd, R., & Davis, M.). (2014). *Home is where we start from: Essays by a psychoanalyst*. W.W. Norton & Company.

Yalom, I. D. (2011). *Staring at the sun: Being at peace with your own mortality*. Little, Brown Book Group.

6

THE HUMAN CONDITION

People are just as wonderful as sunsets if I can let them be. When I look at the sunset, I don't find myself saying, 'Soften the orange a bit on the righthand corner'. . . I don't try to control a sunset. I watch with awe as it unfolds.

Carl Rogers

The ADHD medication had been a salvation for Chris.[1] After years of feeling disconnected and different, they had found a solution. Or so they thought.

Chris had fought long and hard for an appointment with a psychiatrist. The waitlist was months long. The consultation fee had cost the better part of a week's wages. The ongoing costs of stimulant medication an added expense to their already tight budget.

Chris expressed palpable relief at the management of ADHD symptoms. Finally, they could concentrate. Finally, they felt a sense of organisation in life, no longer feeling they were chasing their own tail. Finally, their brain was working as it should. Finally, finally, finally.

They were riding a wave of post-diagnosis euphoria. Like a kid on Christmas morning, ensconced in the wonderment of unwrapped presents and piles of discarded wrapping paper, anticipating the afternoon and long days ahead that would be spent exploring new gifts.

But what goes up, must come down. After a few months of stable mood and better managed anxiety, Chris presented to our session distressed and teary.

It had been a horrible week. Difficult social interactions, a tough time at work, their house was a mess, dishes piled in the sink, kitchen bin overflowing, the dogs hadn't been walked in days. Nothing, they bemoaned, was working as it should.

"I'm pretty sure I have Autism. I've been looking it up online."

"Tell me more," I prompted gently, noticing a piece of paper in their clenched hand.

"It all fits, it's me down to the ground. Every single symptom. Every single one! I saw it on TikTok. It was like looking in a mirror. Then I did a checklist on another website. I scored, like, super high on almost all of the questions."

Chris proceeded to list symptoms of Autism Spectrum Disorder (ASD), citing examples from throughout their life. Chronic anxiety in social situations. Feeling awkward in new

DOI: 10.4324/9781003621645-7

environments. Concentration difficulties at school. Dressing differently from their peers. Loving trivia quizzes. Hating the textures of certain foods. Collecting memorabilia from their favourite bands. Remembering lyrics to obscure songs. Solving sudoku puzzles in record time.

"I've never felt like I've fitted in anywhere. *Anywhere!*" they emphasised, as if realising this for the first time. "I've always been different. I mean, just look at me!" They ran their hand down the side of their body, as if a magician's assistant readying the audience for a big reveal. They pointed to bleached hair, mismatched socks, bright gumboots.

"I don't understand people. They don't understand me. I miss stuff all the time. I misread social cues. I interrupt people. I feel bad about everything all the time. I'm always in my own head. It's horrible!"

I listened. And listened.

"I'm pretty sure I am an AuDHDer."

"A. . . Au. . . can you repeat that for me?"

It was the first time I had heard the term. I often learn sayings and slang from patients; the millennial generation's fondness for the term '100%' to express complete agreement, 'adulting' to describe anything remotely involving responsibility or decision-making, and 'catching feelings' as a kind of shorthand for falling in love. An AuDHDer, Chris explained to me, is a person who identifies as having both Autism and ADHD. A text message to my peer supervision group provided some reassurance that I was not completely out of the loop, with my colleagues also unfamiliar with the term.

Where to now, they asked. Is there medication for this? Do I need to get a formal diagnosis? Back to the psychiatrist? Their voice trailed off as they seemed to be silently considering the expense and likely long wait for another psychiatrist appointment. What does this all mean?

"I don't know what I'm expecting from you. I don't know what you're going to say. Well, maybe I do know what you're likely to say. I was so nervous coming in here today." They continued, before I had a chance to respond to the previous query. "Maybe I want you to tell me, '*this* is it!' But I don't think you're going to do that. I know you're not going to do that. I've been coming here long enough to know that's not how this works. I've spent enough time on this couch to know that is *not* going to happen."

Chris was correct in predicting what I may – or may or not – say. They had brought these thoughts to our session, knowing our conversation was likely to take the form of exploration rather than definition or diagnosis.

The therapy room is a microcosm of the patient's broader world. We draw inferences about patients' functioning and behaviour in their own world through the exchanges in the consulting room. I had not observed any overt signs of neurodiversity in our years of sessions. Chris was punctual to sessions, demonstrated awareness of social cues, promptly paid invoices, gave adequate notice of inability to attend a session, did not interrupt me when speaking, and showed care and consideration of others during brief interactions in the waiting area.

Lack of awareness of time ('time blindness') is one tell-tale sign of neurodiversity. Over time, most patients naturally adhere to sessions being fifty minutes in duration; they pace content and anticipate the finishing time of the session. Neurodiverse patients often do not, missing cues of the imminent end of a session. These may include picking up my diary to schedule the next appointment, glancing at the clock, or, in extreme cases, even standing and gesturing towards the door! Contrary to this, Chris offered agenda items at the beginning of sessions and increasingly took responsibility for time management of sessions.

I reflected this back to them. "It's masking!" they quickly exclaimed. I agreed this is a trait often adopted by autistic people, especially adult females, while overtly wondering if there was something more going on that might account for Chris's distress.

Chris folded the paper neatly and tucked it back inside their bag. They breathed a sigh of relief, as if the list being out of sight meant it was also out of mind.

"I wonder why all this is coming up for you now?"

Chris removed their glasses, held them up to the light, squinting at the smudged lenses.

"I can never get these stupid things clean," they mused. Retrieving a cloth from their pocket, Chris vigorously attacked each blemish on the lens. Apparently satisfied, they replaced their glasses, sighing again as if ready for our conversation to continue.

"Things were going so well. The medication had kicked in. I was on top of stuff. But now it's not working. So maybe it's Autism, not ADHD. Or both? Or is there something else? What else could it be? I *need* an answer to this!"

Their distress was palpable. The sense of urgency and anxiety was not usual for Chris. At least, not usual since commencing stimulant medication.

"I need an answer to this! I've spent so much time and money! I just want an answer!"

I felt their anguish. The inner turmoil of wanting an answer to an unanswerable question. We like to think that life is set, that there is a formula to follow, an equation that will result in one correct answer. Like a series of maths question, marked as right or wrong. Chris's maths worksheet seemed to have transformed from a series of green ticks to a succession of red crosses. Wrong, wrong, wrong. They thought they had figured out the problem. The queries of psychological distress had been put to bed with the rubber stamp of a diagnosis of ADHD.

A scene came into my mind: Chris, in a dusty attic, crouching over an open cardboard box. Desperately searching, trudging through long-forgotten items. The box seems bottomless. Items cascading over the edge, as Chris makes futile efforts to restore some semblance of order. Simultaneously, Chris attempts to reach whatever is buried deep beneath. Chris is searching for something. But what? And what if they found this elusive thing? What would it bring? Meaning, purpose, satisfaction? Maybe all the search would bring was more questions.

How could I help them? I knew I couldn't solve this for them. I couldn't deep-dive into the cardboard box, Mary Poppins style, pulling out a lampshade to illuminate the space, or creating a fantasy world of bright colours and dancing penguins, a world in which everything was miraculously guaranteed to be okay.

But, I could help in the only way I knew how, the one way I know that is often the salve to life's most distressing moments – to listen. To listen without judgement, resisting the temptation to say something cheery or positive. To hold a space for Chris to rifle through those items from that dusty box in the attic, a space to fling out items, throw some back in, leave others untouched.

"We think of Autism," I started gently, aware of the change in tone of my voice in comparison to Chris's rapid-fire listing of symptoms, "as on a spectrum. Many of us fit somewhere on that spectrum. Some people have a few quirky behaviours, others have symptoms that impact their functioning in a much more profound way . . ." My voice trailed off, wanting to give Chris time and space to process this information.

Tears welled in Chris's eyes. We both paused. A silence settled over the room.

"You don't think I have Autism?"

"I'm not sure. I can't tell you that right now, I can't give you an immediate answer. We can work together to explore it. Let's keep talking about it."

Our eyes met. We maintained the gaze.

"But I think what might be more interesting to consider is your curiosity around this, and why this is all emerging for you now."

"You're a human being, Chris," I continued. "A person with many facets, lots of life experiences. You are a reactive, dynamic, wonderful person."

Another long pause. Chris removed their glasses, again checking for smudges. All clear.

"You're a person who has been through a lot. Your mother's death, your sister's addiction. Your dad did his best, but it was tough on all of you. You carried a lot. You were left rudderless, not knowing what was happening. You were untethered. And it seems that sometimes you still feel like that?"

"Untethered – that's the word. I just want something to latch on to. Something to call my own. Why can't I just be a normal person?!"

"I wonder what 'normal' would look like?"

"Just like, being able to do stuff, like other people do. Not mucking stuff up all the time. Not forgetting stuff. Not being such a bloody *idiot* all of the time."

They continued, unprompted.

"Not being that person, that person whose mum has died. That person whose mum is dead. That person whose mum will always be dead! People giving me *that* look, not knowing what to say. Ugh, it's always so awkward. Still is, after all these years."

"You've been through a hell of a lot, Chris. More than most people your age. You've been through real trauma. Trauma shapes us. It's shaped you. You are the result of all these things that have happened to you. You carry it with you. And sometimes it carries you."

"Sometimes it overwhelms me. A lot of the time, it overwhelms me."

Once again, the image of Chris in that dusty attic popped into my mind. Chris, leaping head first into the box of long-lost items. I couldn't find that one magical item for

Chris, I wasn't sure that one magical item even existed. But I could help Chris in their search. I could stand next to them, or throw myself into that box alongside them. Right now, I was standing in that dusty attic with them, arm outstretched, inviting them to reach out and grab on to it, to grab on to me.

"Hello and thanks," heralded the email subject line. The timestamp of 2:13 am gave an indication of the likely course of Chris's rumination following our session the preceding afternoon. Chris apologised for bothering me, continuing on to say that they had been doing a lot of thinking. They had lots to consider, the words attachment and trauma swirling uncomfortably in their mind. Did I have any books I could recommend on this? They thought that might be a good way of avoiding going down the rabbit hole of Dr Google-ing symptoms.

"I'm glad you reached out. You're not bothering me at all," I replied. I recommended a couple of books and reiterated that they were welcome to borrow the books from me during our next appointment. I would put the books aside, ready for collection. A sign of confidence on two fronts. First, Chris would be back, despite our difficult session. Second, I trusted Chris would return the loaned books.

Perhaps Chris would meet the diagnostic criteria for Autism. A screening tool we completed together indicated further assessment may be warranted. Chris, however, chose not to pursue further testing, citing financial and time constraints.

I know these things about Chris, none of which I needed a screening tool to evaluate: Chris is kind, unique, funny, warm, and generous. They have a keen eye for second-hand clothes store bargains. They will never be able to resist stopping to pat a dog. They are a world authority on all things Harry Potter. They would be an asset to any trivia team. They have an infectious laugh, and a wonderfully dark sense of humour. They are true to their word, and always return borrowed books.

A magnificent coastal sunrise emerges from the cool dark of night. Striking colours of orange, pink, and purple. The hues are spilling over hills, slowly illuminating the waves of the ocean as the colour of the water changes from black to blue. The white peaks of the waves glisten with the increasing light.

It is a beautiful sunrise. The sunrise yesterday, however, was arguably more striking — richer tones, dramatic clouds, strobes of light dancing furtively across the sky. I had set my alarm early, hoping to recapture the beauty of that morning. I rolled out of bed, stepping into the chill of the space between the dark of the night and the light of the morning.

But I do not wish for that sunrise instead of this one. I do not wish to change the sunrise, nor do I wish to change Chris. I am watching with awe as they unfold.

NOTE

1 Chris identified as transgender, with preferred pronouns of 'they/them'.

FURTHER READING

Diagnostic and statistical manual of mental disorders: DSM-5 (5th ed. Special ed.). (2017). CBS Publishers & Distributors, Pvt. Ltd.

Flanagan, M. (2016). *On Listening* (Penguin Special). Penguin Books.

Palaniswami, P. (2023, 23 February). Think you've got ADHD? You might not, but you may still need help. *Sydney Morning Herald*. https://www.smh.com.au/lifestyle/health-and-wellness/think-you-ve-got-adhd-you-might-not-but-you-may-still-need-help-20230222-p5cmju.html

Rogers, C. R. (2004). *On becoming a person: A therapist's view of psychotherapy*. Constable.

Schwartz, R. C. (2021). *No bad parts: Healing trauma and restoring wholeness*. Vermilion.

Yalom, I. D. (2017). *The gift of therapy: An open letter to a new generation of therapists and their patients* (reissued). Harper Perennial.

7

SIMILARITY

If you hate a person, you hate something in him that is part of yourself. What isn't part of ourselves doesn't disturb us.

Hermann Hesse

Maya often insisted on reading entire threads of messages verbatim. Her life, she said, was so complicated that reading each word was the only way to accurately convey her experiences. The ubiquity of smartphones seems to have led to an increase of patients reading slabs of text messages or emails aloud in session, and Maya was no exception.

In this instance, 19-year-old Maya was reading a recent text exchange with her mother.

"You are so absorbed in your relationship that you've forgotten everyone and everything else . . ."

My ears pricked up.

"Can you go back to that sentence . . . can you read it again?"

Maya repeated it. I asked whether that message had been written by Maya or her mother. Maya had primarily lived with her mother following her parents' divorce several years earlier. The maternal relationship had been the focus of much of our work, together with her burgeoning relationship with 23-year-old Jacob.

"Me, that bit was from me."

"Oh, I wasn't sure. It sounds like something your mum said to you in another text thread. Am I remembering that correctly?"

"Yeah, I suppose, maybe," she mumbled, not looking up from her phone. Maya swiftly returned to reading verbatim.

"So, Mum wrote, *'you left the heating on all night, the bill is going to be astronomical!'* So, I replied, *'That is not true. It can't have happened because we weren't even there that night! Stop blaming us for stuff that we didn't do!'* Angry emoji, the one with the red face and steam coming from the ears."

By noting the similarity between Maya and her mother, I was attempting to broaden the scope of our conversation. I hoped that moving away from tit-for-tat arguments about specific events and issues, such as heating bills, would move our sessions from

DOI: 10.4324/9781003621645-8

debriefing towards discussing deeper psychological concepts around Maya's experience of the dynamics within her maternal relationship.

"Let's go back to that sentence. *You are so absorbed in your relationship that you've forgotten everyone and everything else.* What do you make of that? Was there something in particular that prompted you to write that?"

"Yeah, Ben. Since she has been seeing him, she's just forgotten about everything and everyone else. Like we don't matter anymore. It's 'Ben this', and 'Ben that', 'blah, blah, blah.'" Maya imitated her mother's voice, using a high-pitched whining tone that sounded more adolescent than maternal.

"It seems like a real shift in your relationship, to feel so distant from her and feel her attention is completely on Ben."

"Yeah, it is like we don't exist now he's around."

Maya again returned to her phone, launching into reading messages with her boyfriend, Jacob, regarding the heater.

Maya was reluctant to spend time away from Jacob. She struggled to sleep without him by her side. She had lost contact with her high school friends, having found she was no longer asked to social events after declining a number of invitations since meeting Jacob. Maya would only attend events to which Jacob was also invited. This caused friction within the family. Notably, Maya was upset by a cousin's refusal to add Jacob to the guestlist of her long-planned wedding. Maya was surprised by her family's stance of understanding the bride's decision, emphasising to Maya that she could survive one evening without Jacob. After much conjecture, Maya declined the solo invitation and did not attend.

Maya often opined that her family did not consider her relationship with Jacob to be serious. They *were* serious, she assured me. Maya and Jacob had recently celebrated their six-month anniversary. Yes, they were young, but age doesn't mean anything, she protested. Neither of them had felt this way before. They knew this was it for both of them, they would be together for the rest of their lives.

A few weeks later, a friend and I were preparing dinner. The easy flow of our friendship had developed over many years. We fell into the natural rhythm of our common cadence – deep and meaningful conversation, discussing the trials and tribulations of parenting, catching up on news about friends and acquaintances.

We had communicated earlier in the day about the meal, both agreeing on an early dinner time to mitigate the chances of 'witching hour' striking our younger children. I superseded her idea of a Mexican meal by saying I was already on my way to the store to buy ingredients for a roast chicken dinner.

I allocated my friend the task of peeling potatoes. She dawdled on this, becoming distracted with preparing drinks and searching for the perfect 'Saturday afternoon cooking' music playlist. I watched as she emptied ice from the tray, debated the merits of lemon or lime twists (finally deciding on lime), measured a shot of gin into each glass, then topped both with sparkling tonic water. I silently took over the task of peeling potatoes.

I suggested she begin on dessert, pointing to the ingredients and recipe I had lined up neatly on the freshly-wiped bench.

"Mum! She won't let me do what I want. She said my idea was silly and she refused to film it! And then she said, 'ugh, you're taking too long', and walked off!"

It was our daughters, running into the kitchen in search of our arbitration.

"Well, she *was*! I let her do the bit with holding the cat and talking about what cats eat . . . but she wanted to say more about it and it was going on for *so* long. It was getting *boring* and we were running out of time!"

My daughter turned on her heel, chin in the air and arms crossed, letting out an audible sigh as she retreated to the nearby sofa.

The argument between our daughters had taken my friend and me by surprise. Up until that point, the two had been seeming to engage in harmonious play. The girls had known each other since infancy, with this playdate the latest in dozens over many years. They had set off into the garden to make a 'documentary' on their iPads about the life of the family cat. Giggling and laughter had abruptly turned to discord, with Louise stomping into the kitchen to air her grievances.

I knew immediately that Louise's recollections were accurate. In that moment, my daughter had been bossy, domineering, impatient. I bristled at this thought, feeling a sense of shame at these aspects of her personality being on display.

Moreover, I saw myself reflected in my daughter. I was also being bossy, domineering, impatient about dinner and its preparation. My delivery had more finesse and less impulsivity than that of my 8-year-old daughter, but there was no denying the similarity in our temperament and behaviour. I was bristling not only at my daughter's behaviour, but the recognition of these shared characteristics of our personalities.

The cat slinked past, oblivious to the fuss to which she was central. My friend and I locked eyes above the fray of the girls' bickering.

"Holy hell," my friend commented, wide-eyed as she took a swill of her drink, "they're the miniature version of us."

Characteristics we dislike in others can teach us a great deal about ourselves.

Arguably, this experience is never richer than between a parent and child. Or, for me and many others, between mother and daughter. There is something cutting and precise about the moment your child reflects your own facial expression, your own tone of voice, a flick of the hair, a roll of the eyes.

"So, I said to her, 'Mum, get a grip!' Seriously, the way she giggles at every joke Ben makes. Like, he's not even funny. She just gushes over him. Even Jacob sees it. He hates it too. They're like two teenagers who can't keep their hands off each other. It's gross. We're like, 'get a room!'"

"Can I share my thoughts about what might be going on here?"

I took Maya's shrug as implicit permission to continue.

"The things that irritate us about others can teach us something about ourselves. Some characteristics or traits of other people can be particularly irritating to us. Sometimes, this is because it reflects a characteristic or trait within ourselves that we may not be particularly fond of."

"I don't get it," Maya replied quickly.

"Your Mum's focus on Ben and her relationship with him annoys you. I wonder if that's because you, yourself, feel a bit unsettled by something about your relationship with Jacob."

Maya's bemused look endured.

"You have said that you and your mum can both be stubborn and hot-headed, especially when firing off text messages to each other. And you've also told me that these things about her annoy you. These annoy you about your mum, but perhaps moreover they annoy you about yourself?"

More bemusement. But at least she wasn't looking at her phone. I had her attention.

"Let's use an example from outside of your family. I'm the cook in my household. I plan the meals, do the shopping, cook the meals. No one else really has a say."

Maya smiled ever so slightly, perhaps happy to have the focus seemingly off her for a moment.

"I was on a weekend away with a few other families. One parent took charge of the kitchen – planned the meals, did the shopping, cooked all the meals. None of us had a say on what we ate, or what time meals were served. They even insisted on doing all the dishes. I felt really annoyed! I wasn't sure why at first. Shouldn't I be relieved to have a break from being in the kitchen?! Then I realised – that parent had taken control of *everything*. I can also be controlling. Sometimes I assume responsibility for things without asking for others' input or opinions. At times, I really dislike that about myself. And seeing those characteristics in that other parent – the way they took control of the kitchen and all the meals – really riled me. I saw a fair bit of myself reflected back at me in that person. And I did not like what I saw."

"Yeah . . . but this is different," Maya shot back.

"Yes, a different situation," I conceded, "but let's look at the broader themes here. Let's focus on why it bothers you, rather than on the he-said-she-said stuff."

I pointed in the direction of Maya's smartphone. She placed it face-down an arm's length away, the furthest distance between Maya and her phone I had witnessed.

"I think there's something about your relationship with Jacob coming up here. You've said that you're absorbed with each other. Obsessed is another word you've used."

"Yeah, like I tell my mum, we're serious. We're going to get married. This is her future son-in-law! You would think she would be a bit nicer to him!"

"You still feel that they are not taking your relationship seriously."

"Yes! And it sucks! I mean, we're not kids any more. We're *adults*, and they need to start treating us like we are. When *we* have kids, I am never going to treat them like they are treating us!"

Maya's contradictory reference to being both an adult and a child seemed to demonstrate her own confusion.

I resisted speaking aloud my line of thought. I was wondering what defined them as adults, wondering who was paying their bills, wondering why neither Maya nor Jacob had jobs nor their driver's licences. The word *entitled* crept into my mind. These two were playing house on someone else's dime. It wasn't a stretch for me to imagine being annoyed should one of my children be acting like Maya. Here, I found myself identifying with Maya's mother.

These were ungenerous and unhelpful thoughts. I was running the risk of edging into territory well worn by Maya's mother, who often reminded Maya that she was living under her roof and needed to respect her rules. With some patients these could be used as challenging statements to show a different perspective. Maya, however, was not one of those patients. This was no time to play devil's advocate.

I made a conscious effort to pull myself away from these thoughts and focus instead on sustaining empathy and positive regard for Maya.

I thought of myself at Maya's age, recalling my boyfriend of the time. I was devoted to him, and he to me. The feeling of superiority that came from being in a serious relationship, the sense of magic and wonderment that came from our mutual adoration. I was enthralled, convinced we would spend the rest of our lives together. (Spoiler alert: I haven't seen that man or thought about him for years. In fact, I can't even recall his surname, which I was once considering taking as my own.) But it would be futile to lecture Maya about my experience of relationships, pointless to share with her the statistics about the longevity of relationships formed in adolescence. If anything, this would likely push Maya to rally harder for her relationship with Jacob, shutting down any possibility that she would share with me any current or future difficulties within it.

Thinking about my own experiences was important, allowing me to better identify with Maya. But I was wary of projecting my own experience of adolescent love and relationships on to her.

"When you say to your mum that she is so absorbed with her relationship that she is letting other stuff slide, I wonder if you're actually talking about yourself a bit, too? I wonder if a part of you is uncomfortable with the idea of your dependence on Jacob? You have said that you've let go of a few things since your relationship began – you dropped your Uni studies, lost contact with your high school friends, you've skipped a few family events, too . . ."

I was concerned that Maya may be becoming dependent on Jacob. At only 19, she seemed to have little in her life outside of the relationship with Jacob. Maya was increasingly isolated from her family and friends, and not pursuing study or employment. She was seemingly prioritising her relationship with Jacob above all else.

"I just want them to take me seriously, to take our relationship seriously! Why does Ben get to stay over every night? He's basically moved in. His stuff is in the bathroom, his toothbrush and his special toothpaste. Of course he needs a special toothpaste. *Ugh*. But Jacob is only allowed to stay two nights a week. So, we have to go between my mum's house and his dad's house for us to spend time together. They spend *every* night together, but she tries to stop *us* doing that."

Maya seemed to understand the concept of what I was saying – that seeing traits in others that we dislike about ourselves can cause us distress. But she was neither ready nor willing to delve further into this topic. I backed away from talking about the notion of similarity.

"What is that like for you, when he's there all the time and even leaves his toothbrush in the bathroom?"

"*And* his toothpaste! It's annoying. I don't want to see his gross toothbrush. Yuk." She rolled her eyes, a palpable look of disgust.

"Just thinking about everything that has happened over the past six months. It seems to have been a real time of change. Your relationship with Jacob becoming more serious, your mum's boyfriend basically moving in. His toothbrush and toothpaste appearing! You and Jacob hopping between houses to spend time together . . ."

"I don't want to be without him. I can't be, it really upsets me when we are apart."

"You come to our sessions on your own. What's it like for you to be here, without Jacob?"

"Yeah, but this is *different*. It's, like, a proper appointment."

Maya's passive 'yes . . . but' response was reminiscent of a child–parent conversation, in which the child acknowledges but quickly dismisses a solution. My own response was designed to encourage Maya to move away from this child–parent dynamic, to one informed by Maya's sense of autonomy and maturity. I was careful to steer away from lecturing Maya, not wanting to entrench a child–parent dynamic in our therapeutic relationship.

"Sure, but give yourself some credit – you travel to and from these appointments on your own, and he's not here with us for this hour every week."

"Yeah, I do. And sometimes I go to the supermarket on the way home."

"Sometimes it's kind of nice to miss someone. Absence makes the heart grow fonder?"

The old adage was lost on Maya. I forged on, thinking better than to explain its meaning.

"You know something that might strengthen your relationship with Jacob even more? Doing things for yourself, and doing things with other people. What are you doing that's just yours? What do you have for yourself?"

While I could see that Maya and Jacob's relationship was certainly intense, I was not sure it was secure. Secure attachment – widely recognised to be the most adaptive and healthy form of attachment – is demonstrated by comfort in spending some time alone or without a significant other, safe in the knowledge that they can be depended on to return. Other forms of attachment include avoidant (characterised by the individual rebuffing others' attempts for contact or connection, as they have experienced rejection of their own attempts for contact or connection), resistant (alert, unsettled, ambivalent or angry response to attempts to comfort), and disorganised (feeling undeserving of care, often resulting from neglect or childhood trauma).

Maya seemed to be showing signs of an anxious attachment. She was preoccupied with the availability and responsiveness of others in her life. A child who is anxious may cling to their parent's leg when left at childcare or kindergarten; in later years, these physical manifestations may be replaced by more internalised forms of fretting.

"Well, nothing really. Coming here. I'm not spending the night without him, if that's what you're going to suggest!"

"I know that it's really important for you to be with Jacob overnight. I wonder what else we could think of? Something just for you."

"I don't know," she responded.

I encouraged her to think for a moment, assuring her there was no rush and no wrong answer.

"I've been meaning to call my friend. The one from high school that I told you about. She's moved out into a share house. I guess I could go over and visit her. It would be nice to see her."

"Sounds like a great idea," I responded, relieved to hear an independent thought, thankful I resisted the temptation of making suggestions.

"Sometimes you bring a take-away coffee into session . . ."

"Oh, should I be bringing you one, too?! I didn't even think of that. What's your order?"

"No, I am always well-caffeinated. Thanks for the kind offer, though!"

It was refreshing to hear Maya consider my perspective. This was an indication that she was thinking of something – anything – beyond herself and Jacob.

"You are welcome to bring a take-away coffee in here, that's no bother at all. But I wonder how it might be for you to arrive for our appointment a little early, say half an hour? And then spend that time having a coffee at the café downstairs, rather than bringing it as a take-away?"

"Yeah, I could do that," Maya sounded confident in her response. "Might take a magazine to read. I really need to spend less time on my phone."

A few sessions later, Maya was recalling an experience with her mother. She relayed a tense interaction that had played out over the past few days. Maya's mother had spoken tersely to Maya and Jacob, assuming the unwashed dishes in the sink belonged to them. In fact, Maya's brother had left the unwashed dishes. Maya was upset about her mum's outburst, thinking her mum could have asked if the dishes were theirs, rather than making an assumption.

"I think one of the reasons it annoyed me so much is that sometimes I can be like that. You know, a bit . . . kind of, reactive. A bit quick to judge, to jump to conclusions."

Maybe, just maybe, something had sunk in from our earlier conversations.

"Oh, that's interesting," I started. "Tell me more about what you noticed."

Most mother-daughter dyads share characteristics. Some are overt and noticeable, such as physical appearance, academic aptitude, or sporting prowess. More covert characteristics are more difficult to notice but are arguably just as impactful.

Our way of being in the world is shaped, in large part, by our early experiences with caregivers and key attachment figures. Intergenerational traits are garnered by both genetic (inherited) and social (environmental) transmission. As a result, our personalities and behaviours will inevitably reflect those involved in our upbringing.

Introspection can be a difficult and emotionally laborious task. It is perhaps understandable then that we resist acknowledging challenging aspects of our own personalities, instead identifying them as 'annoying' in another person. One way of increasing our patience and appreciation of ourselves and others is to notice these shared characteristics, recognising them as neither good nor bad, but instead exploring these aspects and reaching an understanding of their origins and impact.

FURTHER READING

DeYoung, P. A. (2022). *Understanding and treating chronic shame: Healing right brain relational trauma.* Routledge.

Gostečnik, C. (2017). *Relational family therapy: The systemic, interpersonal, and intrapsychic experience.* Routledge.

Jaffe, A. (with Winston, C., Winston, R., & Jung, C. G.). (2011). *Memories, dreams, reflections.* Knopf Doubleday Publishing Group.

Jung, C. G. (2013). *The psychology of the transference.* Taylor and Francis.

Levine, A., & Heller, R. S. F. (2011). *Attached: The new science of adult attachment and how it can help you find – and keep – love* (paperback ed.). Jeremy P. Tarcher.

Schwartz, R. C. (2021). *No bad parts: Healing trauma and restoring wholeness.* Vermilion.

Winnicott, D. W. (1998). *Babies and their mothers.* Addison-Wesley Publishing.

Winnicott, D. W. (with Winnicott, C., Shepherd, R., & Davis, M.). (2014). *Home is where we start from: Essays by a psychoanalyst.* W.W. Norton & Company.

Wolynn, M. (2017). *It didn't start with you: How inherited family trauma shapes who we are and how to end the cycle.* Penguin Books.

Yalom, I. D. (2000). *Momma and the meaning of life: Tales of psychotherapy.* Perennial.

8

THE UNSENT LETTER

When we cannot find a way of telling our story, our story tells us – we dream these
stories, we develop symptoms, or we find ourselves acting in ways we don't understand.

Stephen Grosz

Humans have a peculiar habit of believing their own thoughts. More recently, this seems to
have extended to believing that all thoughts need to be shared. All of our thoughts, all of the
time. Immediate communication and instant gratification. Didn't like the service at a café?
Post a review for friends and strangers alike. Unhappy with your football team's coaching
decisions? You best post it on a forum and argue it out with thousands of other fans.

But a thought is not a fact. And not all thoughts should necessarily be shared.

It may sound paradoxical for a therapist to discourage sharing thoughts and feelings.
That, however, is exactly the therapeutic approach I use with some patients.

"I don't know what to do with these thoughts! I am *so* damn angry with her. So damn
angry with both of them. They're the adults here, *they* are the parents. I'm the kid, they
shouldn't be putting this stuff on me."

Jo had been surprised by the end of her parents' marriage. She had long known the
union was not a happy one, but nevertheless their impending divorce was unexpected.
She thought they would likely live unhappily ever after. The final dissolution of their
relationship was the catalyst for much psychological distress for Jo.

"I know about the affair. I want to tell her that I know about the affair. Who does
she think she is kidding? Her marriage ends and the next day she meets that guy. You
don't just leave a marriage of twenty-five years and then take up with Fabio the next
day. Where did she find him? At the gym. Aha, *right*. Well, if it's that easy to find attractive men, maybe we should all start going to the gym more often! Except, you know,
I'm more of a wine and cheese platter kind of person."

Jo was a delightful woman with whom to work. We quickly established a strong
therapeutic rapport. Easy and free-flowing conversations were aided by a shared
language from the television series *Seinfeld*, together with references and phrases
from mutual favourite authors. "Not that there's anything wrong with that" was

DOI: 10.4324/9781003621645-9

oft-cited to indicate no judgement of others' choices, while references to the egocentric and arguably selfish behaviour of Jerry and his group of friends were used to draw parallels to Jo's experience of her parents' regressed behaviour. Jo reflected that her parents were acting with the immaturity and inelegance of George Costanza during the 'Big Salad' episode.

Jo's father was devastated by the breakdown of the marriage, despite acknowledging long-term difficulties within it. He turned to Jo and her sister for emotional and practical support. Most of the care fell to Jo, with her sister busy with a young family of her own.

"He's never even made himself a meal! How does a man get to fifty-five years of age and not be able to feed himself? Seriously, the man doesn't even know how to boil water. And mum. What's the definition of a mid-life crisis? Because I'm pretty sure she's having one. Like the female version of an old bald guy driving a convertible car with the top down."

"Your mum's behaviour seems especially irritating to you. What do you make of this 'mid-life crisis'?"

"Look, I'm happy for her. I really am. I mean, she seems to have a better love life than me. She's got the glow of a woman who is spending *a lot* of time in bed. Not that there's anything wrong with that! Ugh, I can't even believe I'm talking about my mum and Fabio having sex . . ."

Fabio was Jo's pseudonym for her mother's boyfriend. Unable to bring herself to use his name, 'Fabio' was a homage to his younger age, muscular physique, and flowing blonde locks. The light-hearted references to Fabio provided some levity to our conversations. Jo was adept at using humour as a coping mechanism, both in session and in her everyday life.

"I've been thinking about what you asked me. About my thoughts of when mum actually left the family."

Her mother's slow but steady disengagement from the family had been the focus of much of our work together.

"I always got the feeling she never wanted to be a mum. I don't know why people have children if they don't want them. Children don't have a choice about being born, you know. So, if you bring a kid into this world, you better step up and care for them."

There had been a change to the tone of our sessions. Light-hearted references to her father's culinary ineptitude and mother's sex life replaced with more considered thoughts.

"Your parents' divorce and her starting a new relationship seems the latest in a long list of surprises from your mum," I offered.

The dissolution of her parents' relationship had led to the revelation of long-held family secrets. Her mother's pregnancy with Jo had been unplanned. In Jo's words, the pregnancy precipitated a "good-old fashioned shotgun wedding." The arrival of Jo's younger sister followed a few years later. But the biggest shock was yet to come: Jo's mother had experienced a severe case of 'baby blues', which we would now understand to be postnatal depression. She had been sent to the country for several weeks for 'rest and fresh air' following Jo's birth. Jo was cared for by paternal grandparents during this time of separation.

These revelations had up-ended Jo's image of her family. She began questioning her childhood and family experiences.

"Does it mean she didn't want me? I guess she didn't. She was always a bit flaky. Other mums were baking cakes and packing lunchboxes, we always had lunch orders. I thought it was cool at the time, a special treat every day. She never came on excursions, never helped out for school events. Now I realise it was probably because of her laziness."

"I wonder if part of that could also be attributed to depression, given what we know now?"

"Yes, I can see that now. She did have days in bed, she drank too much . . . it just seemed that she wasn't suited to family life and parenting."

"What was that like for you? What were your experiences of your mum being depressed, of her disengagement from the family?"

"I suppose I became self-sufficient. And I like that about myself. I don't need to rely on her or anyone else. But now I'm being asked to be sufficient not only for myself, but to manage mum and dad's bullshit, too," she sighed.

"You have experienced parentification for a long time. Having to assume responsibility for things that were not appropriate for a child of your age. And your parents are still doing it. In fact, it seems to be increasing. They are looking to you to sort out their financial settlement, relaying messages between the two. You are hearing each make disparaging comments about the other. You are quite literally stuck in the middle."

"Don't get me wrong, we weren't mistreated. We had dinner on the table every night, we weren't walking barefoot through five miles of snow to get to school."

Many adults exploring the impact of their childhood and family speak similar words. They are reluctant to criticise their parents. They are at pains to emphasise the material care received; most were well-dressed, well-fed, taken to swimming lessons and weekend sports. Invariably, they pre-emptively dismiss any notion of physical or sexual abuse.

Most parents, I tell patients, do their best with the resources available to them. None of us are perfect. Parenting is a tough gig. Acknowledging and exploring difficult childhood circumstances or the impact of parents' behaviour or parenting styles need not be a sign of lack of gratitude. Parenting, like life itself, tends to throw all sorts of surprises at us.

"She's taking us all for fools. I need to tell her that I know about the affair. I want to confront her. I *need* to confront her."

Proceedings between Jo's parents had become increasingly acrimonious. Arguments about money, property, even ownership of the family dog.

"I mean, for goodness' sake, Max is geriatric. If they go to court about this stuff, I doubt the dog will even be alive by the time it's all finished!"

Jo seemed to be the parent here, speaking in clear language and citing common sense.

"Maybe your parents are playing out their relationship with you and your sister through ownership of Max? If you two were younger, I guess this is what their custody battle would look like?"

"I'm just thankful that I am old enough that they can't fight over custody of me!"

"Not officially or through the court system, anyway," I added.

"Well, I actually don't think mum would bother to fight for custody of us. She's basically disappeared out of all of our lives. Consumed with her new life, with Fabio, consumed with anything that's not us." Jo shook her head, an indication of disbelief at her mum's disengagement from the family.

"And then yesterday dad asked me how to get divorced. Seriously. He asked *me*, his daughter, how to get divorced. Can the man not use Google? Can he not call a lawyer? So, I looked it up. You can lodge it online these days. An electronic form and a few hundred dollars, and you are no longer married."

Jo again shook her head, a sign of escalating irritation and frustration at her parents.

"He wants me to do it for him. And he wants me to write 'infidelity' as the reason for the divorce. I thought everyone just said 'irreconcilable differences'. Dad seems to think he's in some Hollywood movie, that mum is going to be dragged through court and labelled a scarlet woman and paraded in front of the whole town. Seriously, what's he got to prove? To show the certificate down at the golf club?!"

"It seems he's still really hurting from this. Not being able to get a straight story about when Fabio came on the scene. It seems you're all still confused by that whole sequence of events . . . something just doesn't add up."

"It sure doesn't add up. Maybe if I just help him with the divorce, that will be the end of it. I can print off the forms, fill out some parts of it."

Jo seemed resigned to her father's hopelessness. If she didn't help him, who would? He had been abandoned by his wife, her mother. His world turned upside down. In a way, Jo seemed to have stepped into the role of her mother, caring for him and being turned to for assistance on a variety of tasks, ranging from small to significant.

Our strong therapeutic rapport encouraged me to thrash out issues in a forthright and frank manner. "Jo, you should stay out of this. Tell your dad to get a lawyer to sort out filing the divorce. I think you need to treat your parents as two separate people. I know it's hard to think of them as individuals after so long of them being one unit, but they are no longer married. And you being stuck in the middle of their childish bickering is doing no one any good, least of all you. She is still your mum and he is still your dad. They always will be. But they are not your 'mum and dad' in a collective sense."

"Yes, I know. I know. You're not the first person to tell me this."

"What do you think it is that's holding you back from setting some firmer boundaries?"

"I feel horrible for him. I mean, he's been abandoned. You know, they made a pact to be there for each other. Till death do them part, apparently. Well, they're both very much alive. He isn't equipped for this. He has been left stranded. High and dry. If I'm not there for him, who will be?"

"Sounds like he was completely blindsided by your mum leaving. It came as a real surprise. And the inauspicious circumstances around Fabio. I can understand his confusion and distress. And yours, too."

I continued, wanting to bring the conversation back to Jo. "I wonder if you relate to that feeling your dad seems to be experiencing, the feeling of being abandoned by your mother? She seems a stranger to you both. This new version of your mum, she's so foreign to you both."

"Yep, she's a stranger. I don't even recognise her now. I don't know if it's Botox or something else, she just looks weird! And she doesn't sound like my mum, she doesn't talk like her. She's like a Stepford Wife, but servile to her new boyfriend rather than her husband. It's all so strange."

"Your dad will be okay. Sure, he's a bit hapless. But he will survive. He's got a lot of strengths too – let's not forget he established a very successful company and found a great place to live after the separation. And he has good support around him – friends from the golf club, your uncles, his grandkids. Let your sister and the kids take some of the load off you."

"I guess what you're saying to me is that I need to butt out of his life?"

"Well, yes. That's a more succinct way of putting it!"

"I'm sure there's a relevant *Seinfeld* reference here . . ." Jo mused, before answering her own question, "'Serenity now!'?"

We both laughed.

The beloved Scottish author Ali Smith paid homage to another Scot, Olive Fraser, in her anthology, *Public Library*. Fraser, a poet, was born in Edinburgh in 1909, raised by an aunt after being abandoned as a newborn by her parents, who were estranged from both each other and their daughter. Fraser's distress was compounded by living in the same small town as her parents; incidental meetings were met with indifference, without any recognition or response. The lifelong pain of being an unwanted child permeated much of her writing.

Fraser grew to be a renowned beauty and lively companion. An outstanding student, she attended the universities of Aberdeen and Cambridge to study English. Later stages of her life were marked with mental illness, vagrancy, and ill health. Treatment for schizophrenia impeded her ability to write. Later in life, treatment for hypothyroidism brought relief from chronic depressive symptoms and raised doubt about the earlier diagnosis of schizophrenia. Fraser died isolated and impoverished, her poetry largely unpublished and arguably under-recognised.

Fraser epitomised her experience of maternal abandonment and parental estrangement in her poem, 'The Unwanted Child'. Written long after the death of her parents, just a few years before her own death at the age of 67, Fraser's poem was never read by those responsible for her anguish. This does nothing to diminish its significance. Meaning often lies in expression, rather than reception.

I was the wrong music
The wrong guest for you
When I came through the tundras
And thro' the dew.
Summon'd, tho' unwanted,
Hated, tho' true
I came by golden mountains
To dwell with you.
I took strange Algol with me
And Betelgeuse, but you
Wanted a purse of gold
And interest to accrue.
You could have had them all,
The dust, the glories too,
But I was the wrong music
And why I never knew.

"Have you given any more thought to speaking with your mother? Or, as you said last time, confronting her?"

Jo was not prone to rash decisions. For this I was grateful; it gave us time to work through her thoughts and feelings, providing space for herself without unnecessarily joining the family's warfare.

I shared Olive Fraser's poem and a brief synopsis of her life. Jo wept as I read 'The Unwanted Child'. Tears welled in my own eyes.

I wondered aloud if Jo could consider something similar.

"It seems important to express your thoughts about your parents, especially your mum. And, of course, we can do that in this space. But I wonder what it might be like to also write a letter? An unsent letter, to be specific."

"You don't think I should say these things straight to them?"

"What do you think that may bring?"

"Oh gosh, probably just more arguments, more acrimony, more mud-slinging. And I just don't think I could face them. I can't confront them. Not right now, anyway."

"I wonder if they would even be capable of hearing you, of *really* hearing you? They seem quite self-consumed at the moment."

"That's putting it nicely! They're incapable of hearing me – or anyone else – at the moment. Maybe in the future, but not right now."

"There's benefit in expressing your thoughts about them, but perhaps less benefit in expressing those thoughts directly to them. What matters most is the *expression* of what you have to say. Having a chance to say it can help us clarify ideas. Putting it down on paper, stream of consciousness style, can relieve some of the pressure and distress brought about by the thoughts."

"I'm no Olive Fraser, but I like the idea. I used to do a bit of creative writing at university, it would be nice to get back into it." Jo seemed enthused by the notion of having a channel to express her long-held ruminative thoughts.

We discussed the practicalities of the 'unsent letter'; I emphasised the letter was to remain unsent, while Jo mused the type of notebook that may befit this heady task.

As is often the case with patients to whom I recommend this task, Jo took a few attempts at writing the unsent letter. She deliberated on the task over our next few sessions.

I empathised with Jo about the gravity of writing the unsent letter. Much would be brought to the fore. It may feel unnatural to write a letter focusing on her parents. It may even feel like an act of betrayal. Despite their difficulties, Jo very much loved her parents and craved ongoing relationships with them both.

I gently reminded Jo that while the letter was unsent, she was very welcome to read it aloud in session, when she was ready.

The brilliance of Jo's writing was no surprise. Her quick wit and sharp conversational skills translated seamlessly to the page.

Dear Mum,

The heat this week has been excruciating. I have sought refuge from my stifling apartment in any way possible. Yesterday, I spent the afternoon sitting under the shade of a huge fig tree at Fitzroy Gardens. Its generous canopy provided much-needed relief from the scorching January day.

A petite elderly woman and her daughter approached. A chirpy "hello!" sung in unison towards my direction. So much conveyed in just one word – a greeting, a query as to whether they could intrude upon my solitude, acknowledgement of the heat of the day and the need to shelter under the cool of the tree.

The mother and daughter chatted and giggled for a minute or so while setting up their patch. Lawn chairs, a picnic blanket, a couple of bottles of sparkling water, a packet of potato chips, a stack of books, the day's newspaper.

They silently swapped sections of the newspaper, reading a few headlines aloud. The older lady scribbled letters into the crossword grid. Both looked bemused about a particular clue. Starting with L, ending with E, with a D somewhere in the middle. The younger woman craned her neck to see the newspaper, then clicked her fingers softly and closed her eyes, concentrating and trawling the annals of her mind for long lost information, before exclaiming the 7-letter word. The older woman threw her head back with glee, emphatically writing the letters into the grid.

Pride. The older woman was proud of her daughter.

An immense sadness came over me. What was it like to be praised, to be the focus of your mother's attention?

They moved on quickly. This moment of small celebration – so foreign to me that I watched from a distance like a voyeur, my slightly agape mouth hidden behind a takeaway coffee cup – passed as quickly as it had occurred. The younger woman picked up a book, adjusting her glasses before focusing on the page. The older woman folded the newspaper and placed it next to her, the pen rolling slightly downhill as she placed it atop the paper. She sat quietly, sipping water.

I sat and watched them for longer than I care to admit. I wondered about the lives of these women. They seemed so at ease with each other. Kindness and light. Warmth and comfort. A relationship honed over years. How many conversations – some easy, some no doubt difficult – had they shared? How many newspapers had they read together? How many afternoons had they enjoyed in each other's company?

I imagined their lives. Comfortable but modest homes. A daughter who takes her ageing mother to medical appointments. A pair content to spend this swelter-ing day together, sitting under the cool shade of a beautiful tree. I imagined that in years gone by the older woman would have doted on young grandchildren, the chil-dren of her daughter. The grandmother would have helped with working through the usual foibles and challenges of parenting – feeding, toileting, the tricky teenage years. I imagined her adult grandchildren adoring her now, towering over her phys-ically, reciprocating the love they received.

I mourned that I have never had this. I mourned that I will never have this.

Thoughts of defectiveness set into my mind. The word (the thought, the feeling, the gut-wrenching drop in the pit of my stomach) fell into my mind as if it were a pin placed on a map. "Gotcha now," it seemed to say, burrowing deeper and deeper into my psyche. There must be something about me, something so deeply repulsive, so deeply offensive, that I am not allowed to have whatever it was that that nice mother and daughter have. I don't deserve it. I am undeserving. Undeserving. My place is to sit a few metres back, an observer living vicariously through the everyday interactions of two strangers.

I'm sure they've not given me another thought. Me, the 30-something-year-old woman sitting under a tree with a book and a takeaway coffee. I'm sure they've had countless moments like that since that day. The shared joy of finding the answer to the crossword clue has undoubtedly long since faded. A small moment of time in their lives, insignificant to them, but extraordinary to me.

Maybe I am mourning for a relationship with you, my mother, that never really was. Something we never really had. Whatever it was, it now seems truly over.

Where are you, mum? I don't know how you fill your days. I don't know anything about your life with Fabio. How can your life not involve me and dad, and Anne and the kids? How could you just forget about us like that?

I remember waiting at the school yard gates. The hordes of parents and students quickly dissipated as the minutes passed. The streets crowded with cars just a few moments before were suddenly empty. Where were you, Mum?

I remember watching Saturday morning cartoons on TV. I heard you and dad arguing in the next room. You said that you are going to leave. Will you leave, Mum?

I remember lying in bed, staring at the glow-in-the-dark stars on the ceiling. I heard your footsteps down the hallway, the jingle of your keys, the creak of the door closing, the hum of the motor as the car reversed down the driveway. Where were you going, Mum?

Where are you, mum?

Love always, Jo.

I have had the privilege of hearing many unsent letters to a variety of recipients. But few featured the prescience, clarity, and palpable emotion expressed by Jo.

We sat in silence for a minute or so.

"Jo, may I share my thoughts?"

"Yes, please do!"

"First, your writing is brilliant. You must write! You have a gift, a talent. Keep writing!"

"I actually really enjoyed writing it. I mean, it sounds kind of wrong to say I enjoyed it, given the content, but in a strange way, I did."

"I could certainly sense your commitment to the task, your involvement in it. What was it like to write it, and read it aloud?"

"Much more powerful than I anticipated. I was really emotionally drawn after writing it, slept for a solid ten hours. Which I think might have been just what I needed. Something seems to have lifted though. Things with my parents haven't changed, they are still being painful and difficult. But something about my perspective on it all has shifted."

"And reading it aloud?"

"Well, thanks for listening to it! And thanks for listening to me bang on about my parents for the last however many months! Maybe we should have done that in the first session?!"

"I think you knew when you were ready to write it. It's not something that can be rushed. May I ask, what are you planning on doing with the letter?"

"I'm sure as hell not going to send it. I might add a bit more to it over the next few days. I think I'm going to hold onto it for a little while, until the cooler weather when we light the fireplace. I'll throw the letter in the fire and watch it burn to smithereens. Could be quite cathartic."

The acrimony between Jo's parents continued. Her father managed to lodge the divorce application. The relationship between her mother and Fabio remained strong. Jo ever so slowly warmed to him.

The unsent letter prompted quite a career change for Jo. She is now a published writer. You may have read her work. But one thing that will never be attributed to her is the unsent letter to her mother.

FURTHER READING

Beck, J. S., & Beck, A. T. (1995). *Cognitive therapy: Basics and beyond*. Guilford Press.

Denny, B. (2023, 4 October). Silverchair, take it from a psychologist – rehashing your breakup won't help anything. *The Age*. https://www.theage.com.au/culture/music/silverchair-take-it-from-a-psychologist-rehashing-your-breakup-won-t-help-anything-20231003-p5e9gd.html

Fraser, O. (1989). *The wrong music: The poems of Olive Fraser; 1909–1977* (H. M. Shire, ed.). Canongate.

Grosz, S. (2013). *The examined life: How we lose and find ourselves*. Chatto & Windus.

Morgan, A. (2000). *What is narrative therapy? An easy-to-read introduction*. Dulwich Centre Publications.

Smith, A. (2016). *Public library and other stories*. Penguin Books.

Yalom, I. D. (2000). *Momma and the meaning of life: Tales of psychotherapy*. Perennial.

Young, J. E. (with Klosko, J. S., & Beck, A. T.). (1994). *Reinventing your life: The breakthrough program to end negative behavior . . . and feel great again*. Penguin Publishing Group.

Young, J. E., Klosko, J. S., & Weishaar, M. E. (2007). *Schema therapy: A practitioner's guide*. Guilford Press.

9

ALL WORK AND NO PLAY

I am sometimes driven to the conclusion that boring people need treatment more urgently than mad people.

Carl Jung

The therapist's chair is a place of belonging for me. Like many therapists, my vocation is more than a job; it brings meaning, purpose, a sense of professional and personal identity, and a feeling of belonging with my group of peers.

We all have places to which we belong. That is, if we are lucky enough to find them. I have a few beyond the therapist's chair: my polka-dotted yoga mat, pottering in my vegetable patch, reading in front of a raging open fireplace, watching a movie with my children. For others, it's a buzzing sports stadium, sitting around the family dinner table, being behind the wheel of a sports car on a wide open road, running a marathon, or swimming laps at the local pool.

We identify strongly with our vocations. Workplaces offer a safe, familiar place. A home away from home. For some people, work seems to be the *only* place they experience a sense of belonging. But all work and no play makes Jack a dull boy. Or, in this case, all work and no play was making my patient, Iliana, very boring indeed.

I did not look forward to sessions with Iliana. Sometimes, I dreaded the sessions. An extra coffee would help keep my mind sharp, help keep the ball rolling. Still, the content of our sessions seemed superficial, never moving into the territory of meaningful or therapeutic discussion. It felt impossible to gain any traction.

Each session devolved into discussion of another tedious workplace quandary. I found myself recycling the same tired reflections, reaching for the same analogies, implying the same advice. Iliana was amenable to my suggestions and observations, nodding in agreement with a concept or idea, never querying its meaning or showing any inclination towards deeper thought. She struggled to generate her own ideas despite prompts and leading questions. I found myself doing most of the talking, often breaking my rule of never exceeding the words spoken by a patient during a session.

DOI: 10.4324/9781003621645-10

We were putting out spot fires, never quite able to draw our attention to the raging forest fire that seemed to be underpinning Iliana's distress. With the *content* of our sessions seemingly going nowhere fast, I turned my mind to the *process*. I remembered the words of a colleague: the art of therapy is to simultaneously listen *to* while listening *for*. In other words, it is important to be mindful of both content (what is being said) and process (how it is being said, and what is occurring between the therapist and patient during their conversation).

I had tried to push aside my feelings of boredom. I had tried to caffeinate them away. I had tried to schedule morning rather than afternoon appointments, knowing my mind is sharper in the earlier hours. I had tried to be jovial and good-humoured, perhaps hoping that modelling levity would excavate some buried *joie de vivre* from somewhere deep within Iliana.

I imagined the dynamic between us was similar to Iliana's interactions with other individuals in her life – agreeable, non-combative, avoidant of any confrontation. My experience of Iliana was that she was a nice but altogether underwhelming woman. This was likely also indicative of others' experience of her.

This state of ennui was an uncomfortable feeling. Increasing feelings of guilt about my work with Iliana were the cherry on top of the boredom sundae. From where was this guilt emanating? Iliana seemed content with our sessions; she continued to schedule appointments, was punctual, never late with payment. She was conscientious and kind. Iliana was almost *too nice, too considerate.* I felt I was walking all over Iliana by not providing 'proper therapy'.

At first, I felt I wasn't providing Iliana with a good service, no bang for her buck. Perhaps a bit of imposter syndrome from earlier in my career as a therapist had returned, with the feeling that I couldn't figure this person out, that I couldn't help her. Then I put it on her – our inept connection must be due to her deficits. There was no *oomph* to Iliana. She was beige, bland, boring.

Finally, I accepted my feelings of boredom. No longer trying to turn these feelings away, I decided to work with the feelings of boredom rather than try to obliterate them. I realised these feelings were not a contraindication of the direction of therapy. Rather, they were exactly where the therapy needed to be focused.

Iliana identified strongly with her role as a customer service representative for a major bank. In her role at a call-centre, she receiving inbound calls from bank customers querying credit card transactions. Iliana was at the front line of this work, answering initial telephone calls from customers, collecting information, then diverting the call to an appropriate service. Her long-held ambition of working as a bank teller had been stymied by the mass closure of bricks-and-mortar bank branches and the colossal movement towards online banking.

Work played a central and increasingly prominent role in Iliana's life. She spoke of the bank with a sense of ownership and responsibility above that of her role, as indicated by her frequent use of collective language such as "we" and "our." Iliana was perfectionistic about her work. Turning up excessively early for shifts was an antidote for her fear of running late. She expressed annoyance at co-workers who she viewed as "slack" and lacking commitment to the bank. Iliana was baffled by the high staff turnover at the call-centre, musing that a better job could not be found. Iliana had become increasingly fixated on the bank, visiting branches, learning about its history, and closely following any news stories about the bank.

The high regard in which Iliana held the bank seemed neither reciprocated nor appreciated. Leave requests were often denied by management without explanation. Infrequent appeals to colleagues for shift swaps would also be left unanswered, despite Iliana dutifully picking up others' shifts and covering leave. She had been denied promotion several times, watching as colleagues rose through the ranks. Iliana was excluded and left behind.

Iliana was reminiscent of a woman I had met years earlier. Sandy, a friend of a friend, worked at Disney World in Florida. She facilitated our trip to the theme park with just a few days' notice, despite knowing us only through a mutual acquaintance. This tenuous social connection did nothing to dampen her enthusiasm for our visit and the hospitality afforded to us. We enjoyed complimentary entrance to the park, discounted accommodation at a brand-new hotel, and, perhaps best of all, a pass that allowed us to jump the queue for any ride.

Sandy insisted on chaperoning us around Disney World, despite it being her day off. She gleefully described every detail of the theme park. Did you know that there is a Mickey Mouse symbol embedded in the structure of each ride? Did you know that the Swiss Family Treehouse weighs 200 tonnes? Did you know that the design of Disney World's 'Main Street USA' is based on Walt's hometown in Missouri? (Apparently Sandy was on first name basis with Mr Disney.) Did you know that staff are referred to as 'cast members'? Did you know that there is a mammoth network of underground tunnels beneath Disney World, right under our feet?!

No, Sandy, I didn't know any of those mildly interesting facts. I am not a Disney aficionado. I just wanted to wander around the park, have my photo taken with Mickey and Minnie, and . . . well, that was actually all I wanted to do.

Sandy sure had drunk the Disney Kool-Aid. Her own identity seemed inextricably intertwined with Disney. Despite spending the whole day with Sandy, I knew everything about Disney World but little about her. She was protective of the Disney brand and its reputation, and obviously unimpressed when my friend queried the creepier side of life at a theme park – do you ever catch couples in the throes of passion on a ride, is it true the underground tunnels are also used to transport the bodies of guests who have died, is Walt Disney really cryogenically frozen?

I thought I knew what to expect from Disney World. The one thing I didn't anticipate was being jaded and a little bored of it. But somehow Sandy had managed to bring more than a tinge of tedium to the Happiest Place on Earth™.

"I mean, I just can't believe we did that. I can't believe it happened. I'm so embarrassed, so ashamed that we did that."

The bank had dominated news headlines that week, with the revelation of deceased customers being charged ongoing fees. The scandal had been preceded by hefty interest rate rises, prompting speculation and widespread disapproval about the bank's record profits and the staggeringly high salaries and bonuses paid to its CEO and board members. This had been a challenging time for the bank. By extension, this had also been a challenging time for Iliana.

Bottom lip quivering, Iliana was on the precipice of tears but doing her utmost to maintain a calm disposition. I thought of the contrast between Iliana and the bank's CEO. Slick-haired and shiny-skinned, the CEO had fronted various press conferences that week. Cool and confident, he seemed unfazed by the dozens of microphones stabbing the air in front of him. Carefully scripted words and vague phrases provided a cursory statement of facts but steered well clear of any admission of guilt.

That very day, a national newspaper ran a cartoon with a caricature of the shiny and slick CEO. He was surrounded by brimstone and fire, complete with devil horns, a smarmy smile, and literal dollar signs in his eyes.

Iliana was quick to defend the CEO. Her flat affect had given way to an animated expression I had not seen before. "He works hard. *Really* hard. Can you imagine having all that responsibility? It is not an easy job! We do the best to look out for our customers. We're all devastated by everything that has happened."

Iliana's sense of collectivism seemed to have strengthened in the face of this time of adversity for the bank. It seemed that Iliana wanted to protect it; if the bank failed, she would not only lose her job, but her place of belonging.

"How are you experiencing this, in your role at the call-centre?"

"I know our customers are having a tough time of it. It's really horrible for them."

"Yes, it's a very difficult time for many people. But how are *you* experiencing this? How is this impacting *you*?"

"Oh, I suppose I never really thought about it like that. We're all working for good outcomes for the bank. We're the bank, we're part of the team. It's important for us to all stick together."

But Iliana didn't seem to be part of any team. There didn't seem to be a team around her. She was working hard for the bank, taking the worries of work home with her, expressing empathy for a CEO who seemed to show little regard for anyone or anything else.

I wondered what drove Iliana's overidentification with her role at the bank. Any threat to its credibility or stability – such as that of the current scandal – saw Iliana dig in her heels even deeper. She wanted to protect the entity of the bank. A threat to it was a threat to her.

In a later session, I made a concerted effort to steer the conversation away from work.

"How have you been going with the things we talked about last time? Any luck with following up on that book club? Or the gym membership, did you take up that new membership offer you saw advertised?"

"Oh, I haven't had a chance. Things have been so busy with work, especially with all this stuff around the interest rates and charges to deceased customers . . ." A shake of the head and roll of the eyes expressed her ongoing dismay at the growing scandal.

I started to feel impatient. A sense of annoyance setting in. More talk of the bank, interest rates, and dead customers. Tedious, tiresome, repetitive, bland, dreary. Boring. I was bored. My threshold for more bank talk was in imminent danger of being breached, just as it had been hearing the umpteenth fact about Disney World all those years earlier.

"I wonder how much of that is within your control? These are big issues, influenced by worldwide events and people who are way above our pay grade."

"I feel like it's all my responsibility. When I talk to the customers on the phone, I'm responsible to them. They have horrible things happen to them, one I spoke to yesterday had thousands of dollars defrauded, spent on cigarettes and alcohol by a random guy in some place called Albuquerque! Apparently that's somewhere in America. Unbelievable! I mean, how much can one person smoke and drink?!"

This seemed almost exciting to Iliana. Intrigued by the life of a drunken, chain-smoking mystery man in a far-off country. I guessed I wasn't the first person to hear the Albuquerque saga, nor would I be the last.

"The customers whose calls you answer are lucky to land with you. You always go above and beyond. You bring an important sense of humanity to the bank, a real human element to what must be a difficult time for these customers."

We had talked about these interactions before, focusing on strategies to manage Iliana's reaction to difficult phone calls. Some customers were rude and abrupt, distressed and annoyed about credit card issues. Iliana tended to take their insults about the bank personally, dwelling on conversations with customers long after her shift was over.

Distress and rumination seemed the consequence of Iliana's inability to separate any part of her identity or self from the bank. Customers' comments about the bank being "bloody hopeless" and "woefully inept" were a blow to her own already deflated self-esteem. She heard their words as *"you* are hopeless," *"you* are woefully inept."

"How much of this is actually your responsibility? The bank is a huge, multi-national company, with thousands of employees . . . you're one person in a huge corporate system."

I feared I might have said too much, pushed the point too far and too soon. Iliana's obsession with working for the bank was dysfunctional and unhealthy at times, but its centrality to her life was undeniably important. The fixation had developed for a reason. Removing this structure could devastate Iliana. She seemed to have little else in her life, and her efforts to increase activity and joy in other areas had not come to any fruition. Undermining Iliana's ideal image of the bank and the importance of her role within it would likely lead to feelings of devastation and further loneliness. I was reminded of a parable of an empty house my supervisor had once cited: it is not enough to cast an unclean spirit out of a person, an empty house is a target for other even more evil spirits.

"I suppose I can't really control anything . . ."

I was trying to tread lightly. Iliana's ego was fragile. She was vulnerable to any perceived criticism. A wrong step here could cause a rupture in our therapeutic relationship, jeopardising not only her engagement with sessions but potentially her overall wellbeing.

"I think you can! You have some control of the experience the customer has with you on the phone. And you always try your absolute best at that. And we've spoken before about ways you can attempt to control your thoughts and rumination about work. You *cannot* control everything else about that customer's interaction with the bank, or how their credit card issue might or might not be resolved."

Iliana nodded. I was unsure whether this indicated genuine resonance, or was a sign of her usual agreeableness.

"You do a good job, Iliana. A great job. I know how committed you are to the bank and to its customers. But I wonder what cost this is having on you? It seems that sometimes the great work you do is not recognised . . . the leave requests left unanswered, your disappointment about not being promoted to the management role . . ."

Iliana had great difficulty acknowledging and expressing her experiences of unfair treatment, such as when her leave requests were denied without explanation. At the core of this seemed to be shame and embarrassment at being treated unfairly by a workplace to which she gave so much of herself. I was always mindful during our sessions to not further shame or embarrass Iliana.

I saw Iliana being walked over. The bank did not treat her with respect or fairness, much as they were accused of treating their customers – deceased or living – without respect or fairness. I felt defensive and protective of Iliana, wanting to be her advocate. I could see the good in her, a good that was being taken advantage of by the behemoth banking organisation.

At times I felt frustrated with Iliana's inability or unwillingness to stand up for herself. Her passivity provided a sharp contrast to my temperament and sense of volition.

Iliana had latched onto the bank as a place of belonging. She seemed intent on maintaining this narrative, despite increasing evidence of the bank's dirty dealings.

I discussed Iliana with my supervisor. I told him of the guilt I felt as I expressed my frustration at her passivity, lack of psychological thinking, and our perceived lack of therapeutic progress.

"Sometimes I dread our sessions, I need an extra coffee for fear of nodding off! Am I an unkind therapist? I feel like I am a horrible therapist, a horrible person!"

"Oh, Bianca! You're not horrible! You know that. But it seems you *are* struggling to experience empathy for Iliana. She is very different from you – you are a strong-willed and busy person. You don't let the grass grow under your feet, that's for sure. But something about Iliana hits a nerve for you, there's something about her that gets right up your nose . . . because there are parts of her that *are* similar to you."

"Do you think so? I can't see any similarities between us. We're really chalk and cheese!"

"You know what it's like to put your faith in a system and have it fall apart around you. You know that feeling of being deeply connected to a structure that enlarged your life and brought meaning and purpose, but did not always recognise your value and hard work. You don't have to tell Iliana *your* story, but you can use *your* experience to understand *her* experience. You share the experience of being walked over, of people taking advantage of your charity. You share the experience of having been committed to a dysfunctional system. You share the experience of, at times, having been pathologically accommodating to it."

The much-loved American poet Mary Oliver died during the time I was working with Iliana. Oliver was known for her beautiful prose, inspired by her wonderment of the natural world. Although Oliver rarely wrote about people, her work somehow encapsulates the human experience and the human condition.

I recalled a line from one of Oliver's best-known poems, 'The Summer Day'. In it, Oliver reflects on the meaning of the life of a grasshopper, which she observed to move with purpose and grace, despite its minuscule status and short lifespan. The poem concludes with an eloquent existential query:

Tell me, what is it you plan to do
With your one wild and precious life?

I wanted to implore Iliana to grab life with both hands, to see the vast world outside of the bank, to not waste any one moment of her wild and precious life. Look, I wanted to shake her, the immortal Mary Oliver is dead! She has re-joined the earth, drifted away like one of the autumn leaves about which she wrote so beautifully.

We are all going to die! None of us have very long at all! Don't put all your energy into the bank. Stop lining the shareholders' pockets, stop inflating the already over-sized ego of the slimy, veneer-teethed CEO! Stop allowing them to take advantage of your charity.

"I'm just so upset. I don't know what to do. It's my dad's sixtieth birthday. I requested leave months ago. We're going away for four nights. The accommodation is already booked. Everyone is coming, the whole family. My brothers and sisters, my grandparents. I'll be the only one not there."

Excluded. Let down. Again.

Iliana spoke of a close family, a happy childhood. As the youngest daughter in a sibship of four, Iliana remained the last child living at home. She spoke of missing the comradery and activity of having older siblings at home. Similar to connections with work colleagues, she seemed to be the family member making the most effort to increase engagement and maintain contact with her siblings. Iliana was particularly distressed by a belated birthday message from her brother; she would never forget a family member's birthday.

Iliana has experienced feelings of rejection in other areas of her life, including siblings drifting away and moving forward in their lives without her. I was careful to not further evoke feelings of rejection, while being simultaneously aware of the impact of my boredom and tedium on my capacity to feel an empathic connection with Iliana.

"Everything I do for them. I cover every shift. I cover for everyone I never turn down a shift. I work overtime. I can't remember the last time I had a sick day. And this is really the only thing I've ever asked for. It's been the only thing I've really needed from them."

A chasm had emerged between Iliana and the bank. Finally, a glimpse of Iliana, an ever so slight separation from her identity as an employee.

Iliana was experiencing a conflict, an ultimate clash between the two central objects in her life. This struggle could not be easily reconciled. It seemed that something would have to give. It was one or the other of the two systems to which Iliana was most loyal – the bank or her family. She had experienced rejection and disconnection from both. But still, for Iliana blood remains thicker than water.

It seemed that Iliana had now been pushed too far by the bank. Finally, Iliana was expressing her needs. I wanted to capture this, to encourage more expression about a topic other than the bank.

"Tell me more about your dad's birthday."

"We've been planning it for years. It's hard to get everyone together. It's really important to him. It's important to me, to everyone. I don't want to miss out."

"Nor should you miss out! You deserve to go, to spend that time with your family and celebrate your dad's birthday. Your family is important to you, this event is important to you. Important to your whole family!"

"100 percent! It is really important!"

"You're an exemplary employee. You've been nothing but loyal to the bank, especially with everything that's been happening lately. You are a good person working in a difficult place."

"I suppose I do try to take the moral high ground, to bring some kind of good to that place."

"Yes, and it seems that's exhausting! You're always on the watch for ways to help customers, to make sure the bank's reputation is upheld. But it's time to prioritise yourself. Time to find some more balance. Take that trip. Celebrate with your family."

Iliana nodded with enthusiasm.

"The bank will survive. You are valuable to the bank, you are a wonderful employee, but none of us are indispensable to any organisation. Do not let them take advantage of your charity."

I wish I could say that Iliana strode out of our session, submitted her resignation to the bank, enjoyed a fabulous holiday with her family to celebrate her father's birthday, and embarked on a new chapter of her life. I wish I could say that she never looked back, that she never again let anyone – whether a corporation or an individual – take advantage of her kindness and charity.

The reality is, change was much slower. Trepidation soon tempered Iliana's buoyed confidence about pushing for leave and joining the family holiday. She returned to the passive position, defending the bank's actions, and expressing renewed apprehension about requesting leave for the holiday.

This was difficult for Iliana. She was facing a true conundrum – jeopardising her belonging at the bank, without a clear path forward or another place of belonging in which to land. It takes a good deal of ego strength to depart a place when there is no certain way forward.

But, eventually, Iliana did join her family for the holiday to celebrate her father's birthday. She delighted in the company of her parents and siblings. She continued to work at the bank, but was able to implement and maintain firmer boundaries around her role and position. She joined a book club, where after a slow start she made friends with like-minded people. The gym membership started with a flurry of regular exercise. But as is the case for many people who take out a gym membership, the enthusiasm did not last. Iliana called the gym and cancelled the direct debit for her membership. This was despite feeling bad for leaving, worrying about the financial position of the gym and its owners. Iliana did not let them take advantage of her charity.

FURTHER READING

DeYoung, P. A. (2022). *Understanding and treating chronic shame: Healing right brain relational trauma.* Routledge.

Hackney, H. L., & Cormier, S. (2009). *The professional counselor: A process guide to helping.* Merrill.

Jung, C. G. (with Shamdasani, S., Peck, J., & Kyburz, M.). (2012). *The Red Book: A reader's edition* (1st ed.). W. W. Norton & Company.

Oliver, M. (2012). *House of light.* Beacon Press.

Schwartz, R. C. (2021). *No bad parts: Healing trauma and restoring wholeness.* Vermilion.

Yalom, I. D. (2017). *The gift of therapy: An open letter to a new generation of therapists and their patients* (reissued). Harper Perennial.

10

JEALOUSY IS A CURSE

Even so my bloody thoughts with violent pace
Shall ne'er look back, ne'er ebb to humble love.

Othello

I've known about you and Justin for a while now. It just hurts me that you couldn't tell the truth about it.

You must be leaving really early for work these days. 6 am! Your car wasn't in the driveway. Got something to tell me?!

My, you were up early this morning . . . wasn't even daylight!

Having fun?

William Shakespeare wrote of Othello's jealousy in his eponymic play. The character of Othello is conflicted and complex. A scorned army colleague, Iago, manipulates Othello to believe his wife, Desdemona, has been unfaithful. Scraps of information are taken as evidence of Desdemona's deceit. Othello's own insecurities make him a prime target for Iago's manipulation. Othello sees no other option but to murder Desdemona, explaining this ultimate act as a result of loving too much, while not being able to love wisely. In the final analysis, susceptibility to jealousy and suggestibility are revealed as his tragic flaws.

It is after Shakespeare's tragic character that the colloquial term for morbid jealousy, Othello syndrome, is named. This rare psychiatric disorder is equal parts fascinating and terrifying. Othello syndrome is a type of paranoid delusional jealousy. Primarily affecting males, it is characterised by obsessive jealousy of a romantic partner and false beliefs of infidelity. This disorder is typically seen as one aspect of a more complex delusional system. It often co-occurs with other conditions such as mood disorders and personality disorders.

Being the focus of another's obsessive thoughts about infidelity represents an incredibly difficult and unenviable position. As the tale of Desdemona illustrates, it can also be a dangerous position. Othello syndrome may be the precipitant to stalking, harassment, violence, and, in some cases, homicide.

DOI: 10.4324/9781003621645-11

You are pathetic. Just PATHETIC.
You are underhanded and contrived . . .
YOU MUST AND WILL BE HELD ACCOUNTABLE.

"Nicholas, 62-year-old male, second admission. Diagnoses of major depressive disorder, morbid jealousy. Nick has not responded to medication. Depression appears treatment resistant. Visits from his wife, Margaret, were suspended due to Nick's increased irritability and escalation of verbal abuse. First ECT session scheduled for this afternoon."

I was a trainee therapist, completing an internship at an acute psychiatric hospital. The daily case conference offered a précis of patients currently admitted to the ward. The meeting provided a space to discuss matters related to patients, such as diagnosis, medication, and treatment planning. Such meetings are typically overseen by a consultant psychiatrist, with contributions from psychologists, nurses, and other allied health staff members.

Patients' conditions were wide-ranging: psychosis, anorexia nervosa, personality disorders, depression, severe trichotillomania (compulsive hair pulling), post-traumatic stress disorder (PTSD), and self-harming behaviour. Most of the patients on the locked ward were involuntary, meaning they had been deemed at that time to be unable to make decisions regarding their own welfare and treatment.

My time on the ward was a steep learning curve. It was the clinical equivalent of being a kid in a candy shop. Up until that time, I had only read about many of these conditions in textbooks. So much to learn, not only from my supervisors, but from patients themselves.

"Bianca, good opportunity for you to observe ECT. Meet us outside the treatment room at 2 pm."

"Sure, thanks." I readily agreed with the psychiatrist, despite my propensity towards fainting at the sight of blood and general queasiness at the thought of any medical procedure.

I was, of course, familiar with the diagnosis of major depressive disorder. Commonly referred to as depression, major depressive disorder is diagnosed when a patient has experienced two or more episodes of depression. It is a high-prevalence disorder, meaning it is experienced by a high number of individuals in the general population.

However, I had never heard of 'morbid jealousy'. I retreated to the office, in search of the *DSM*, a book which lists psychiatric diagnoses and their symptoms. It was high on the bookshelf, far out of my reach. I grabbed a chair and balanced precariously, retrieving the heavy diagnostic bible. I was keen to understand the condition that appeared to be assumed knowledge during the case conference.

The pages of the *DSM* were tabbed with someone else's fluorescent Post-it notes. I thought of my own copy of the hefty tome, with Post-it notes and pencil scribbles marking important sections. As postgraduate students we studied the *DSM-IV* (now updated to the fifth edition) in meticulous detail, preparing for exams in which we were assessed on our ability to diagnose fictional patients with one of hundreds of conditions. I was retrospectively relieved that 'morbid jealousy' had not featured in my exam!

Perusal of the *DSM* informed me that 'delusional disorder – jealous type' was a low-prevalence disorder, usually experienced by males with a previous diagnosis of a mood disorder or psychotic disorder. The disorder is covered under the broader diagnostic umbrella of delusional disorders. In reading this, I followed a rule that I developed during my training and continue to adhere to today: when feeling overwhelmed or confused by diagnosis and classification of disorders, look first to the broader diagnostic category, rather than the intricate details of the disorder. As I now say to my supervisees: when in doubt, zoom out!

> *Through your own stupidity and selfishness you have put me in this position.*
> *Disgusted in you.*
> *You've been lying to me.*
> *Once again, you have lied to me. I cannot say it more clearly than that.*

Nick was the epitome of misery. Dressed in stained tracksuit pants and an oversized t-shirt, his demeanour was reminiscent of Eeyore on his saddest day. Nick moped around the ward, unable to sit still for any longer than a few minutes. Frustrated at the television show broadcasting in the shared common area, Nick stood up abruptly, slamming the door upon his exit.

Nick's access to telephone calls had been restricted. He was compelled to call Margaret dozens of times each day, such was his obsession with thoughts of her infidelity. Nick would repeat the accusations of infidelity during their telephone conversations. He begged her to be honest with him, to come clean about her years-long affairs. He would interrogate her about the paternity of their children, singling out features of the children's appearances he deemed to be evidence of Margaret's dalliances with other men. In his most distressed moments, Nick would threaten to kill her, followed by himself.

Margaret frequently visited Nick on the ward, bringing a thermos of coffee and a tin of home-made biscuits. She had a smile for everyone, offering biscuits to staff and thanking them profusely for their care of Nick. I found it hard to relate to Margaret. My naïve, trainee therapist self was full of theoretical knowledge, but I was still accruing experience of life itself. How do women find themselves in those situations? Why would such a nice woman ever marry someone like Nick? Why does she even want to visit him, with home-made biscuits, nonetheless? Why does she answer his phone calls, knowing the inevitable bluster and abuse that would ensue? Why doesn't she leave? For goodness' sake, why doesn't she just leave?!

> *You are such a coward. Stand by your actions.*
> *Thanks to your behaviour and choices your life is going to be shit going forward.*
> *You have lied to me on quite a few things to this point. So kinda don't believe you.*
> *In fact, I don't. :)*

I managed to stay conscious during Nick's ECT procedure. (Hint, to combat nausea and the inclination to faint: sit, don't stand; choose a point to focus on, don't look away; press your tongue to the roof of your mouth.)

Electroconvulsive treatment (ECT) is a procedure in which controlled electric currents are passed through the brain. It impacts the brain's activity, and is known to provide effective and fast relief of depressive and psychotic symptoms. Patients typically have a course of several ECT sessions over a number of weeks or months.

Nick was sedated prior to the procedure. He looked peaceful, as if enjoying the forced intermission from the persistent thoughts about Margaret. I wondered if this was the soft, gentle Nick with whom Margaret was familiar. The man she fell in love with, married, with whom she had children and built a life. This contrast prompted me, for the first time, to think of the distress Margaret and Nick's other family members and loved ones likely experienced as a result of his illness. I found myself hoping that ECT would be an effective treatment for Nick. More was at stake than Nick's wellbeing; the ripple effect of an individual experiencing a psychiatric illness, such as a delusional disorder, is significant and far-reaching.

A nurse attached several electrodes to Nick's scalp, mostly concentrated on his forehead. A mouthguard was placed to protect his teeth from damage. The psychiatrist tweaked the controls as if turning a dial on an old-fashioned radio transmitter. Nick's body jolted as the electric currents were activated. The convulsions increased as the higher voltage was administered, his body spasming for half a minute or so.

Twenty minutes on, the procedure was complete. The thrashing movements settled into stillness. Nick was rolled onto his side, vital signs checked, and taken to a recovery bay.

I saw Nick the following day, strolling cheerfully around the ward. His dysthymia and irritability replaced with a slight smile and mild-mannered interactions. I marvelled at the efficacy and efficiency of ECT, thankful for the opportunity to re-write my thinking of it being an outdated and barbaric treatment.

> *I'm starting to think you are fibbing to me!*
> *I do have a HUGE issue with being lied to.*
> *Either tell me the truth now and we can work out a way to approach this . . . or lie to me and jeopardise yourself.*

"We may as well be honest with each other. I'm only here because the lawyer said it would be a good idea before I'm due at court."

The tall, broad-shouldered man had not yet taken a seat before making the definitive statement. His loose-fitting Bintang singlet revealed lobster-red sunburnt shoulders. Faded football shorts and a flimsy pair of flip-flops completed his outfit.

Together with therapeutic rapport, patients' willingness to participate in treatment is a significant predictor of optimal treatment outcomes. Brian had already let me know that he was anything but a willing participant in therapy. In the words of a previous supervisor, I anticipated Brian was likely to be a 'therapy hater'. Doubtful, cynical of the potential benefits of therapy, and likely to disengage with little forewarning.

Many forensic patients present to treatment for a reason not of their own volition. That is, individuals who have had involvement with the criminal justice system may be mandated to attend treatment by a court order or community treatment order. Some may attend at the behest of a lawyer, in anticipation of a court appearance.

I ushered Brian further into the room, encouraging him to take a seat. Sheepishly, he handed me a pile of papers: letters from his lawyer and referring doctor, and a crumpled and stained stapled document that I immediately recognised to be a court-issued family violence order.

I quickly scanned through the paperwork as Brian settled into his seat. The order prohibited Brian from making any contact with his estranged wife, including not going within 50 metres of her or their marital home. Similar conditions had been imposed during Brian's relationship with his former partner, from whom he was also estranged. The GP letter outlined a diagnosis of delusional jealousy, together with Brian's objective of reconciling with his estranged wife. Further details included heavy alcohol consumption (approximately twelve standard drinks per day), non-compliance with anti-depressant medication, and previous incarceration for family violence.

I looked up from the collection of papers. Brian was whistling quietly to himself, glancing around the room.

"Where shall we start today, Brian?"

My usual practice is to begin sessions with a broad question, regardless of pre-existing knowledge about the patient. Hearing the patient's experience in their own words usually gives more prescient information than even the most detailed referral.

"I may as well get straight to it," Brian sighed, as if about to launch into a well-rehearsed speech.

"Me wife is cheating on me. Val. She's done the dirty on me. A bloke from her work. I knew it was going on for a while. Then she came home late from some work party. Said it was a farewell party, but – get this – no one has left her work! I'm not stupid. She took me for a fool. A *fool*!"

Despite the distressing content, Brian's voice was cheery and his smile broad. This incongruent affect struck me as odd.

"So, I threatened to kill him," Brian continued, in a light-hearted and whimsical tone. "He bloody well deserved it. The hide of them both, outright lying to me like that. And I would have, too right I would have, if the police didn't get to me first. Val called the cops, said I had hit her and slashed her tyres."

He smiled again. A beguiling look. I theorised Brian to be a man accustomed to being in a position of intimidating people, especially women. I knew my initial interactions with Brian would shape our further work together. As such, I was aiming to achieve a balance between establishing some kind of rapport while being mindful to neither collude with him nor dismiss or belittle his perceived position of power (Seu, 1998).

"It sounds like a lot has been happening, Brian."

My understatement was intentional. I wanted to maintain a sense of calm in our session, especially knowing that Brian may be quick to anger. Mindful of my own safety, I scanned the room and was reassured to know I was seated closest to the door. I was also reassured with the knowledge that I could likely run faster than an overweight and severely sunburnt middle-aged man.

"Could we take a step back for a moment? I'm interested to hear about your life at home, and then we can talk a little more about what's brought you in today."

Brian provided a surprisingly succinct overview of his life. This was clearly not his first session with a mental health clinician, nor the first time he had been asked to recall details of his family and background.

His life had been punctuated by transience and ruined chances. A difficult childhood and unhappy family home had been marked by a violent relationship between his parents, with Brian stating that his mother "gave as good as she got." School studies gave way to an adolescence of petty crime, leading to several stints in juvenile boys' homes. In later years, employment in the construction industry had been hampered by claims of bullying and theft.

Several romantic relationships had soured after accusations of violence, excessive alcohol consumption, and financial strain. A brief marriage produced two children; Brian was estranged from his former wife and children.

Val, Brian pined, was special. He knew she was different, right from the moment their eyes locked across the pool table of the local pub. Things were meant to be different with her, he sighed. But she too had betrayed him. Unbelievable, he muttered, shaking his head in disbelief. But he was willing to give her a second chance, if only she would come clean with him. All would be forgiven, if only she would admit what was going on between her and that dweeb of a bloke at work.

"Val wants the intervention order lifted, of course," Brian continued with a confidence usually reserved for white male politicians. "But the bloody cops and the bloody court won't have it. She regrets ever getting the bloody thing."

In fact, the police had applied for the intervention order on Val's behalf. Val had made no application for the order, nor was she able to withdraw or modify an order that had been taken out on her behalf.

"Can you tell me a bit more about Val?"

And off he went. The Val floodgates had opened. It was difficult to contain Brian, so eager was he to recall every detail of his shared history with Val. A flurry of fast-paced and tangential information, jumping from banal and trivial facts to intimate and intricate tales.

Val was the woman of his dreams. He recalled their first meeting, first kiss, first night together. Her favourite food was pizza, but it had to be from their special place in town. Their table was always reserved for them, no one else dared sit in their booth. A small wedding, attended by just one witness. They weren't showy, didn't need a big ceremony. Brian and Val had it all. Beautiful house. A boat. Both loved their dogs, treated them as the children they never had. He missed the dogs, wanted to see the dogs. His voice changed tone as he stated she had no right to take the dogs from him. Brian made no mention of the former wife and children from whom he was estranged.

"It sounds like things have not been as cheery lately . . ." I suggested, seizing the brief opportunity to intervene in Brian's flight of ideas.

"Ever since she took up with that bloke . . ."

"Yes, can you tell me more about your thoughts on that?" I was careful to not collude with Brian. I was asking him about his *thoughts* on Val's infidelity, rather than endorsing his views as correct or factual.

Brian repeated the 'evidence' of Val's infidelity: late night drinks, a lift home from work with the co-worker in question, Val wearing a new perfume ("obviously to impress him"), and slow replies to Brian's slew of messages during her workday.

I was wary of challenging Brian's assumptions. A delusion is a rigid belief that is held despite evidence to the contrary. I could present Brian with logical reasons for all of Val's actions, but this would be futile at this early juncture of treatment, likely inducing hostility towards me and perhaps leading to disengagement from sessions.

Instead, I asked Brian what he would like to achieve from our sessions together, acknowledging that part of the reason for his attendance was to pre-empt the possibility of court-ordered treatment.

"Well, I want Val back. So, I need you to get rid of this bloody court order."

You are a disgraceful, shameless human being . . .

   I can deal with being disappointed in you, but cannot deal with not being able to trust you.

"The bloody police are trying to keep us apart. Val wants me back. Val wants us back together at home, but the police won't have any of it."

"What's that like for you, Brian?"

"Well, it's bloody frustrating."

Brian's neck and face were now the colour of his lobster-red shoulders. I was unsure whether this was the result of agitation and frustration, or further exposure to the summer sun since our last session.

Several sessions with Brian had provided enough content to inform the beginnings of my thinking regarding a formulation. A middle-aged man with a history of being both a victim and a perpetrator of family violence. A tendency towards paranoid and delusional thinking, with a current fixation on unfounded ideas regarding his wife's infidelity. Difficulty in managing and challenging such beliefs was compounded by heavy alcohol use and non-compliance with medication.

By this time, I had realised that my work with Brian was likely to be short term. Brian was only interested in attending sessions for the advantage he perceived it may bring him in contesting the intervention order. Any shift in Brian's delusional beliefs would come only from his own personal investment in long-term intensive treatment. With this knowledge, I came to view our treatment goals and the purpose of our sessions in a different way. I was aiming to keep Brian engaged in sessions until his court date or such time that his care could be handed over to a more appropriate service. During this time, I could continue to monitor any change in his condition and provide ongoing assessment of risk to himself and others.

> *Gutted by who you've become.*
> *I'm quite pissed over your deception.*
> *Give me the truth.*

"She's not returning my calls. Val has gone cold on me. After all this, Val's gone cold on me. Of all people, for fuck's sake," he sighed.

Brian's usual gusto and bravado was absent, replaced with a sort of reverence that I had not before witnessed from him. I strained to hear his quietened and mumbled voice, as he repeated murmurings about Val turning cold.

I expected bitterness and scorn, vitriolic descriptions of Val, swearing and raised voice. Instead, Brian seemed deflated. A sadness, a crumbling of stature, an abrupt puncture to his seemingly unshakable confidence in his relationship with Val.

Perhaps some of the reality of his situation had finally become clear. Brian continued to express delusional ideas regarding Val's infidelity, but the tangible impact of his actions seemed to be hitting home.

In that moment, I saw a vulnerable man stripped of his armour. Perhaps he was realising some truths about his life and relationships. The blame for the intervention order and subsequent events were not simply the remit of the police. Instead, Brian seemed to be beginning to realise that the order intended to protect Val did, in fact, seem to be now supported by Val.

I thought of Val's safety. Brian seemed distressed, but not agitated. His usual bluster and bravado had been replaced by melancholy. I was concerned that this change in tone – from a fierce warrior fighting for his woman to a resigned and scorned man relegated to the position of estranged husband – could precipitate a change in his approach and behaviour towards Val.

"When was your last contact with Val? Do you know her whereabouts?"

"Nah, she's blocked my number. Got a message from her sister telling me not to bother calling, reckons that would be stalking her. Ha! Says the locks at home have been changed."

I agreed with Brian that there did indeed seem to be a change in Val's communication.

"What's that like for you, this change from Val in her communication?"

"Bloody dreadful. Bloody, bloody dreadful. Don't worry, I'm not going to do anything stupid, to myself or anyone else."

I guessed Brian was accustomed to risk assessments. I pushed a little further, asking of his plans after our session ("the pub"), his access to any weapons ("just me fists, love"), and his desire to see Val ("I never want to see that two-faced bitch again, for as long as I live").

I recorded in my notes Brian's denial of risk to himself or Val. As I hit 'save' on the file I asked myself a question that I often ponder while conducting risk assessments – should the worst imaginable happen, how would my notes and rationale be viewed in a Coroner's Court? I was confident that I had conducted a thorough risk assessment, but was I truly confident that Brian did not represent a risk to himself or others?

Keep in mind that I might just be a little more aware of the things than you realise.
I'm just so sick of the lies and I think it reflects very badly on you.
You have proven yourself to be the biggest liar and manipulator I've ever known.

"I've met someone. Mel. She's *fantastic*. She's unlike any other woman I've ever met before. Unique. Met her at the caravan park. In the laundromat. Of all places to meet the love of your life, *the laundromat!* Ha!"

Brian was laughing to himself. Like a teenager in love, his high-pitched and fast-paced voice one of infatuation.

"So, no bother about the intervention order stuff now. See ya later, Val!" He offered an exaggerated wave, as if farewelling a distant aeroplane from the observation deck at an airport. "And don't let the door hit you on the way out!"

"Now we have Mel, instead of Val . . .?" My statement sounded more sarcastic than I had intended it to. Brian's boisterous mood, however, was not hampered by my slight *faux pas.*

"She's fantastic. Bright, a good looker. Owns her own site at the caravan park. I've moved in there, no rent to pay on my own now."

"Gosh, it sounds like things are happening quickly!"

"Why wait? I love her, she loves me. We're not getting any younger . . ."

"And where does Val fit into all of this?"

"Oh, *screw* Val! She can do whatever she wants now! I could not care less! COULD. NOT. CARE. LESS."

And with that, Brian was gone. I reported back to his GP and lawyer, stating that Brian had disengaged from treatment, citing a change in his circumstances.

I quietly hoped Mel might also see the correspondence.

My problem is you withheld information from me instead of being honest. Now I have to start considering whether or not you are telling me the truth about everything else.
BIG GAME CHANGER.
I'm done. And so disappointed in who you have become.
YOUR ARROGANCE WILL COST YOU.

Margaret and Val are by no means alone as victims of family violence. In Australia, at least 100 women are killed each year at the hands of their domestic partner.

While I never saw Val, I imagined her as distinct from Margaret. Diverse backgrounds, and disparate socio-economic and family circumstances. Regardless, both had experienced family violence.

Family violence can happen to anyone. The impetus for such violence is varied. Not all will be as a consequence of a delusional disorder. The story of each survivor of family violence – and of those who do not survive to tell their story – is distinct. But the result is the same: behaviour that intimidates, threatens, and terrifies.

> *You need to see someone and get your head straight.*
> *It's all there in black and white . . . evident and true.*
> *Tell yourself whatever you need to, won't ultimately make any difference.*
> *I've seen you do horrible things . . . it pains me.*

Imagine, for a moment, receiving the text messages scattered throughout this chapter. Reams and reams of venomous bile. False accusations, nasty names, outlandish claims. Constantly berated with a 'truth' that in no way reconciles with reality.

Trepidation every time your phone beeps. There is no point blocking the man's number. He will buy a 'burner phone' or revert to email messages.

Ignoring the messages is taken as admittance of guilt. Responding, however, fans the flames of the narcissistic behaviour, likely inciting a further diatribe. Worse still, ignoring contact may prompt him to turn up on your doorstep, intent on delivering his messages verbally. Or physically. Look what you've made him do! A double bind for victims of violence and abuse. The ultimate Catch-22.

Many readers do not need to imagine this scenario. They have lived it. Many continue to live it.

I do not need to imagine this scenario. I have lived it. I was the recipient of those text messages, and hundreds more just like it.

Those messages offer a salient reminder of an almost unbearable time in my life. How did I recover? The only way I know how. Therapy.

FURTHER READING

Behary, W. T. (2021). *Disarming the narcissist: Surviving and thriving with the self-absorbed* (3rd ed.). New Harbinger Publications.

Diagnostic and statistical manual of mental disorders: DSM-5 (5th ed. Special ed.). (2017). CBS Publishers & Distributors, Pvt. Ltd.

Gabbard, G. O. (2005). *Psychodynamic psychiatry in clinical practice* (4th ed). American Psychiatric Pub.

Hill, J. (2021). *See what you made me do: Power, control and domestic abuse.* Black Inc.

Kesey, K. (2008). *One flew over the cuckoo's nest.* Penguin.

McWilliams, N. (1999). *Psychoanalytical case formulation.* Guilford Press.

Oyebode, F. (2021). *Psychopathology of rare and unusual syndromes* (1st ed.). Cambridge University Press. https://doi.org/10.1017/9781108591652

Seu, I. B. (ed.). (1998). *Feminism and psychotherapy: Reflections on contemporary theories and practices.* Sage.

Shakespeare, W. (with Wells, S.). (2015). *Othello* (new ed.). Penguin Classics.

Skorobogatov, A. (with Yazhbin Chavasse, I.). (2023). *Russian Gothic* (1st ed.). Old Street Publishing.

Sperry, L. (2016). *Handbook of diagnosis and treatment of DSM-5 personality disorders: Assessment, case conceptualization, and treatment* (3rd ed.). Routledge.

White, G. L., & Mullen, P. E. (1989). *Jealousy: Theory, research and clinical strategies.* Guilford Press.

INDEX

Abandonment 9, 11, 62, 77

Anxiety 40, 46, 49, 50, 59, 61

Attachment style 1, 24, 25, 26, 29, 63, 70, 71

Attention Deficit Hyperactive Disorder (ADHD) 1, 3, 59, 60, 61

AuDHD 60

Autism Spectrum Disorder (ASD) 59, 60, 61, 62, 63

Boundaries 20, 22, 28, 76, 91

Breadcrumbing 33

Chris (case study) 59–64

Cognitive-behavioural therapy 16

Countertransference 4, 40, 43, 46, 47

Defence mechanism 4, 36, 51

Delusions 15, 16, 93, 95, 96, 97, 99, 100, 101

Denial 3, 4, 33, 35, 36, 41

Depressive disorder 40, 41, 75, 94

Diagnostic and Statistical Manual (DSM) 2, 16, 94, 95

Disney World 85

Ego 22, 28, 39, 44, 74, 88, 89, 91

Electro convulsive therapy (ECT) 94, 96

Emotional deprivation 20, 27

Empathy 8, 14, 51, 69, 86, 88, 89

Envy 14, 17, 44

Estrangement 11, 53, 54

Existential psychotherapy 1, 4, 49, 50, 89

Family therapy 54–56

Family violence 4, 46, 97, 99, 101

Feminist perspective 42, 43

Formulation 39, 42, 50, 53, 99

Fraser, O. 77–79

Freud, S. 2, 14, 27

Grief 1, 3, 4, 13–14, 16, 36, 57

Grosz, S. 73

Hannah (case study) 31–37

Harris, S. 19

Hemingway, E. 45

Hesse, H. 65

Idealising 42, 44

Identity 21, 40, 85, 87, 90

Iliana (case study) 83–91

Isabelle (case study) 40–47

Jealousy 3, 12, 94, 97 *see also* morbid jealousy

Jo (case study) 73–82

John (case study) 8–18

Jung, C. 7, 12, 14, 83

Kierkegaard, S. 49

Kubrick, S. 31

Lee (case study) 49-64

Limerence 20

Love bombing 32

Luke (case study) 19-29

Magical thinking 15–16

Masking 61

Maya (case study) 66–72

Morbid jealousy 93–102 *see also* Othello syndrome

Narcissism 1, 24, 28, 29, 102

Nicholas and Brian (case study) 93–102

Oliver, M. 89

One Flew Over the Cuckoo's Nest 2

Othello syndrome *see* morbid jealousy

Palliative care 49–58

Panic 40, 50, 52

Parentification 40, 75

Paucity mindset 8-9, 51

Perinatal depression 41, 75

Perinatal mental health 4, 41

Personality disorder 3, 19, 93, 94

Post-traumatic stress disorder (PTSD) 16, 94

Primary maternal preoccupation 41

Professional dilemma 22

Projection 15, 32, 43, 45, 47, 69

Regressed behaviour 50, 53, 74

Repetition compulsion 4, 24

Risk assessment 28, 100–101

Rogers, C. 59

Schizophrenia 77

Seinfeld 74, 77

Self-diagnosis 1, 60

Self-disclosure 49

Self-sabotage 25, 26

Shakespeare, W. 94

Shame 3, 11, 15, 28, 67, 88, 99

Similarity 66–72

Smith, A. 77

SSRI medication 40

Synchronicity 7–18

Therapeutic rapport 9, 12, 16, 40, 43, 50, 54, 73, 76, 96, 97

Therapeutic rupture 9, 40, 56, 88

Toxicity 15-17

Transference 4, 43

Trauma 11, 50, 51-52, 55, 62-63

Unsent letter 74, 78–81

Vulnerability 13, 27, 29, 40, 52, 57, 88, 100

Winnicott, D. 41

Yalom, I. 17, 22, 33